How to Think Your Way to Thin

The Lies We Tell Ourselves About Weight Loss

By Robert D. Kintigh

First Edition

Introduction

The time has come to throw away everything you have been taught about weight loss and healthy living. Being fit is not about being skinny and healthy living is not about eating lettuce. Weight loss is accomplished in the mind and I want to show you how you are going to lose weight from your couch if that is what you desire. How to Think Your Way to Thin starts now!

Dieting sucks and exercising is hell and as I lost **105 pounds** using my mind working behind a desk 10-14 hours a day I realized I found something everyone needs. I tried every diet and worked out every day all to end up right back where I started from every time. I was tired of the diet roller coaster and I really had no time to spend hours at a gym. I needed something different that would fit my schedule.

My weight gain came with many excuses along the way. I was big boned was a favorite of mine as well as I was too busy all the time so I grabbed the food I could when I was out and about. I could lose weight if I wanted to but, I just don't want to should have a familiar ring to it as I used it frequently. The mental weight loss training in this book demands that you throw away any excuses as well as stress and anything that will store fat in your body from over burdening yourself.

How to Think Your Way to Thin is designed to help anyone (like you and me) lose weight by harnessing that power you hold in your mind. Do you know how awesome you can really be? Your friends and family will be amazed by what you begin to do as you transform into a slender, healthier person and your attitude will not only greatly improve but become incredible optimistic and positive.

Do you know how you ended up with the weight you currently have? Do you know what it will take to remove the weight you currently have? How long did it take to put that weight on? All of these are great questions because I want to get you thinking about what it will take to remove the weight and understand why you are not at your ideal weight because you do not want to repeat the past so it is paramount to understand and answer these questions.

I will guarantee you that if you will follow what I have for you in this book that you will lose more weight than you ever have before. This is not a diet book and this is not about exercise. Those things are great but, they are the typical path that everyone takes in weight loss. I am taking you down a new path and a new idea that has obvious tremendous benefits.

I bet you are already asking the question how your body can lose weight if you do not exercise or diet. I will not give away any secrets just yet but, I want you to know that it is more than possible to accomplish. I am living proof and so have others I have trained. Your mind is in charge of weight loss and good health and not food and not exercise.

I would urge you to get ready to burn that belly fat and clean out the closet because we are going to blow your mind away with mental weight loss. This is cutting edge stuff and I have what you need. I have the change you desire. I have the program you need to think your way to thin. I have made every effort to give you the best information available and I know what it takes to lose weight mentally. If at any time you feel like this is not for you then I urge you to look at the front cover of this book because it will affirm that you can do this. I would love to hear from you as you think your way to thin.

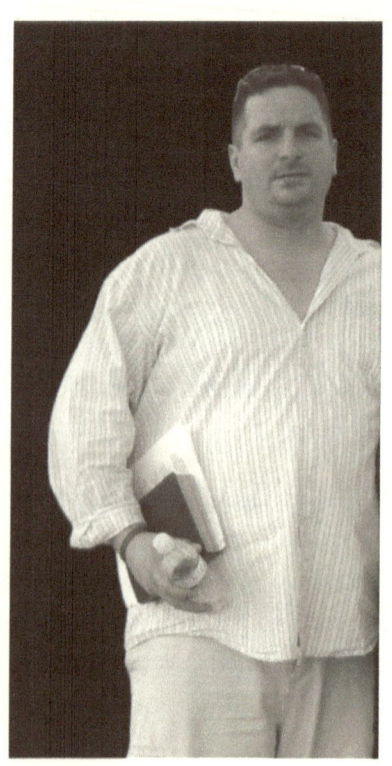

Disclaimer

Every effort has been made to keep everything in this book accurate, honest and without any hype. The author is in no way guaranteeing any specific results and although there have been successful cases with this philosophy and techniques, it is in no way implied you will have the same results. The author is also not a doctor or nutrionist and because of that you should consult a doctor or nutrionist for your own wellbeing.

Nothing in this book is meant to harm you in any way but, only you know what is best for you. Be smart and make sure that you do not put yourself in harm at any time. This is a book about health and losing weight and because of this nature your health is the most important aspect. You should always live a healthy life style and take care of your body.

This book is about utilizing more of your brain power and as long as you are of sound mind, it is my opinion that you can be successful in what I am teaching. I do not know every person or your situation so I cannot say that this is 100% successful for everyone that tries it. Proceed on your own free will.

Why this disclaimer? The Federal Government wants to make sure that there is no trickery involved, false claims or anything that could be misleading. My program has not been evaluated by any government agency. If you proceed in purchasing this book or any subsequent program then you are doing so on your own free will.

Nothing in this book is easy or meant to seem easy. Every person is different and we do not know you so it is up to you to determine if this program is easy or not. We do express that everything in this book is potentially a successful strategy and can be utilized by anyone at any time.

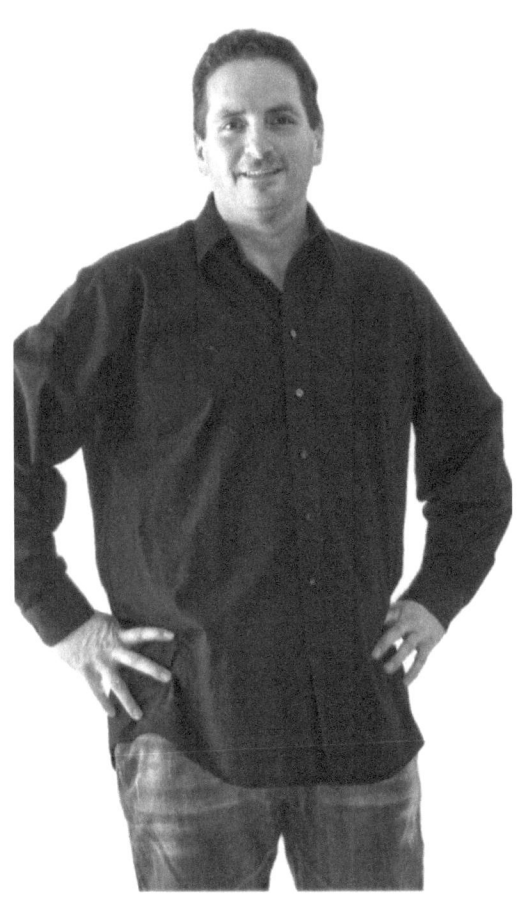

Copyright

Pick Up Other Books by This Author

The Lies We Tell Ourselves

Introduction to Employee Behavior Modification

The Lies We Tell Ourselves Workbook

Small Business Marketing 101

Networking Your Way to Profits

The Mobile App Revolution

Personal Growth in the Work Place

Sales Tips 101 for Future Top Salespeople

On the Run – How to Find Your Runaway Teen

Performance Based Rewards

Mindset – The Power of Your Thoughts

STOP!

Join our newsletter and mailing list and get a ton of great personal growth and development items! Huge value all for the price of FREE as our way of saying thank you!

JOIN OUR NEWSLETTER HERE

www.truthmastery.com

http://www.truthmastery.com/How-to-Think-Your-Way-to-Thin-Weight-Loss-Book-and-Program.html

Table of Contents

Copyright

Dedication

I dedicate this book to people who have struggled to lose weight for a long time. I dedicate this book to anyone who struggles to feel healthy and live with passion and energy. I dedicate this book to people who believe that weight loss is about dieting, exercising and eating salads every day. I dedicate this book to you champion because today is a new day!

I have been an athlete most of my life and I always believed that I was in good shape because I was always working out, eating healthy and playing sports. I was in great shape and did not have a weight issue. Then one day I stopped being that athlete, became a successful entrepreneur and suddenly was overweight. Okay, it did not suddenly just happen one day because fat builds over time and pants get let out as we put on more weight but, it certainly felt like it was over night.

Have you ever had that light bulb moment happen to you? I know you have because everyone has had this happen and that happened with me as all of a sudden it became the answer became clear to me; I was in shape not because I was an athlete per say. I was in shape and healthy because of the way I thought and acted. I had a stellar mindset and knew what I needed to do and how I had to program my mind in order to be successful.

Why do so many people get weight loss wrong? The focus is all wrong and most do not really understand why they can't lose weight. Everything I write about in my books is not dedicated to the super human people of this world. I am an average person and I focus on other normal, average people who can use a helping hand or a leg up. I want to help you who are misinformed and want way more for their life. So this book is for you and I want you to enjoy it and change your life from it!

The Beginning

In December of 2006 I lost my mother to Heart failure, diabetes and kidney failure. It was a blow to everything that I loved and I was in a hole I was not sure that I could get out of (partly because I was so fat – sorry couldn't resist). I loved my mother and she was always the rock I needed to keep me grounded, honest and working on the man I wanted to become. My mother meant so much to me and I felt like I had very little left inside of me as I laid her down to rest.

In February 2007 I could not get out of bed. My entire life up to this point I had always sprung out of bed with passion, enthusiasm and now, I was lucky to fall out of bed. On the morning of my birthday that year in mid-February I had a doctor's appointment scheduled. I had made an appointment for a physical to see if there was anything wrong with me. I did not ask for it to be scheduled on my birthday it was given to me that way. I always say God scheduled it for me even if the nurse's name was Michelle that I spoke with.

I went in for my appointment at 8:30 a.m. the day of my birthday and the first thing they did was weigh me in. The nurse could not get an accurate reading on my weight of the back. I think she was stunned I was over 300 pounds as she kept trying to make two something work. I told her I was over 300 and then she found the level out mark.

Next the doctor came in and I explained to him what was going on with me. After listening for a while and checking me out, he sent me down for a blood test and said they would call me later with any results for a follow up appointment.

I took the blood test and like all of my other birthdays I went out for a day of fun, food and drink. I went shopping; I ate a big juicy burger and had some drinks with my friends. I was living it up and had forgotten about the doctor's appointment from earlier that day. Then around five o'clock I received a call from the doctor's office. The Doctor's nurse called me to have me come back in first thing in the morning.

When I hung up the phone I have to be honest I was worried. It is never good when you go into the doctor first thing in the morning, take a blood test and by the afternoon they are calling you back for first thing in the morning. I was struggling to get out of bed and now I am going to find out why I suppose.

That next morning when I arrived for my appointment I was tired and run down and was very stressed out. I was worrying all night which I am sure was detrimental to me. When the doctor came into my room I was stunned at what he started to tell me.

He said, "Mr. Kintigh, you are 336 pounds and that is a lot of weight to be carrying around and if there were no other problems that would be enough for anyone to get tired and run down and deteriorate their health. Your blood sugar level is 458 which are terrible and very unhealthy. You are Type II Diabetic and we need to get you on some medicine right away." I could feel his sense of urgency and my stress levels rising

The Doctor went on to tell me, "This medicine will give you some immediate relief and you should start to feel more energy come back as well as you should start to feel a whole lot better." I was sitting there in the office stunned, shocked and embarrassed. As I looked down at my stomach he pointed to it and said, "this is what kills most men. That bulge is deadly and the weight you are carrying is very deadly as well."

I am a positive type of guy and always have been. I focus on the challenging and positive and what I want in my life but, somewhere I missed focusing on the right weight I should have been at. I left out of the doctor's office with 4 prescriptions and a heavy heart (no pun intended). I was in bad shape and had to do something about it as soon as I could.

What did I do about it? As you read on you are going to discover everything that I tried and finally accomplished but, what I ended up succeeding at is the basis for this entire book and program.

You have been told so many lies about weight loss, living with being diabetic or other illnesses in this world I think it is time to set things straight (in my opinion). If you are tired of being sick and tired and if you are tired of being overweight then the time has come to dispel the rumors, learn a new way of living and start to open up the power of your mind.

Think Your Way to Thin will only work if you apply it and live it and most importantly, believe in it. The world has lied to you enough so do not lie to yourself any further about how to lose weight or live healthy.

I promise you that what is in this book works no matter how fat or unhealthy you are. I promise it works no matter how sick or ill you may be because the best medicine in the world is already inside of you.

While we are at it, I want to also make something clear as well and that is you need to answer to a higher calling. Faith is a powerful healer and for me I have the luxury to be grounded by God as a Christian. You have your choice of worship and I am not saying that you must believe in what I do but, I know it is extremely important to be of faith, morals and values.

Why is it that diets never work? Why does exercise get old and frustrating? How come some lose weight easily while most suffer a bloated misery? I will give you all of these answers and solutions as we continue on but, what you have to be clear about upfront is that in order to be pretty on the outside, you must cleanse and pretty up the inside. Most people fail no matter what they do because of the ugliness and lack of spirituality inside of their hearts, minds and bodies.

God created a perfect temple called the human body and we do not respect it as we should. We need to repair the work that was started and run our bodies and minds like they were intended as close as we can. I am helping you to unlock a secret that really should have never been a secret to any of us. All of the magic in life has been around us the whole time.

I am so excited to be writing this book and delivering it to you because it is one of the coolest things I have ever figured out in life and I have learned some pretty cool stuff. My hope is that I relay this information to you in a way that has you saying that you get it and you can make it happen because of how I laid it out.

Why this will work for you is that you have tried everything and it all has been painful and frustrating. You have tried rearranging your life, dieting, exercising, and obsessing on what you can't eat and what you want to eat. You are unhappy with the way that you feel and you are ready to go about weight loss and your attitude in a new way.

The time has come to dive into how to think your way to thin works so that you can get yourself to the best place you could ever imagine. Be prepared to open your mind up and change a lot of thoughts that you have been harboring. From this point forward we will change the way we look at food, life, thoughts and how we look at our bodies.

I believe in you and your abilities. I believe in me and the knowledge I have for you. I believe that the mind is the most powerful force in this universe and I believe that you will learn how to harness more of its power in order to begin a powerful transformation in your life.

I know some of the things I will talk about in this book will sound a bit crazy at times and I would not blame you for thinking I am a bit crazy but, I hope that you will give everything I have for you the best chance possible because my story is real and my weight loss is a fact and my body is proof that it works.

The Lies We Tell Ourselves Intro

In August of 2012 I completed my first book called The Lies We Tell Ourselves which is a story of my life and some tough lessons that I learned along the way. This book is a very personal account of my life and how I over came so much along the way even against all odds. The concept of The Lies We Tell Ourselves book is a great foundation for this book you are reading and the two combined have immense power for your life. What does the title of the book mean and how can it impact your life in a positive way?

The main idea behind the book is that the biggest harm we do in our own life is that we constantly lie to ourselves and take on stuff that is not healthy for us. If we tell ourselves we are fat then we will believe we are fat and soon enough we will end up becoming fat. The mind is a powerful element.

So where does my first book tie into this book? Truthfully my first book has everything to do with this book because thinking your way to thin is all about harnessing the power of your brain and if your life is in total chaos and turmoil and if you are not happy and productive, then losing weight is going to be tough no matter what you do.

The Lies We Tell Ourselves is a book about mindset and pushing through no matter how bad you believe your situation is. My father was a bad man, I came from a broken home, and we were not well off and on and on. I know that attitude and mindset determines everything because I have lived it myself and have seen it in so many others as well.

My first book has done very well and I believe with the addition of How to Think Your Way to Thin I will help shed light on what the human spirit is capable of and what power our brains hold for us. I believe these two books alone will drastically change so many lives because the messages are simple, real and extremely powerful. I am an average person trying to do extraordinary things in this world and my hope is to gather as many people like you and me and march all of us successfully down the road of life.

Writing these types of books has been very insightful for me and I hope they will help you as well. I am very passionate about what I write and teach and I know that what I offer works but, in order for them to help you we have to remove limiting beliefs, false ideas and train your mind to kick in to a higher gear.

Now that I have introduced you to both concepts and my books, let's jump into How to Think Your Way to Thin and get our minds and bodies ready for a major transformation. I promise you this will be an interesting journey, mind blowing ideas, eye opening techniques and ideas that will have you thinking like never before! It is my honor to go on this journey with you and no matter how long you have struggled with your weight or your mindset; I know we can become successful together!

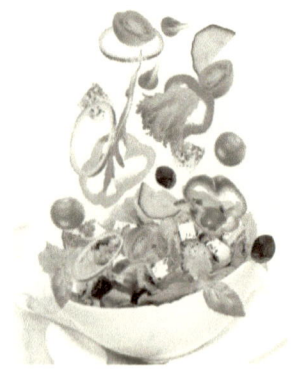

Chapter 1 – How to Think Your Way to Thin

If you don't do what's best for your body, you're the one who comes up on the short end. ~*Julius Erving*

When I started out on my weight loss journey I had a number of ideas of how I was going to accomplish weight loss. I was going to go on a diet and cut out the foods I loved because they were unhealthy I was told. I was going to work out every day until I could barely stand. I was going to lose 20 pounds a month and get back to healthy quick. The ideas I had where ideas that may have been great for the twenty year old me but, the thirty five year old me had different thoughts if I would have listened to them initially because deep down inside I knew I was in trouble.

It was spring time 2007 and I set out to do what I had done so many times when I was younger and that was to hit the gym, get busy being physical and pound away the fat. I had done this my whole life to stay in shape and lose weight so what was going to be the big deal this time?

To understand how crazy this idea was I suggest that you take a ride down to the local Home Depot or Lowes or whatever you have in your town, go to the cement isle and find a 100 pound bag of concrete and try and pick it up and just walk around the store with it for 10 minutes or so.

Let me tell you what is going to start to happen quickly besides just having your clothes get all dirty. As you carry around all of this weight you are going to get tired real quick and your joints are going to first start to ache and then they will begin to throb. Your back will become sore and then progress to feeling very tired and then to a state of aggravated pain and tiredness and advancing to throbbing pain.

There is more that will come your way but, I believe that I am drawing the best picture for you that I can. I was carrying around more than that bag of concrete and it was killing me fast. Maybe you are smaller and are carrying around less weight but it is all conducive to our situation and body type.

So back to my stupid ideas! I started off hitting the gym and working out hard. I was going five to six times a week. I was also playing softball and taking walks. It became a seven day a week affair and I was getting stronger and bulkier. The pounds started to fall off as well yet not quick enough because remember the concrete story a few minutes ago? The pain was beginning to progress.

As I started my exercise program I also started the dirty four letter word as well d-i-e-t. This is a disgusting word in my opinion when it is used in this context because who loves a diet? No one does and because of that it is a death sentence from the very beginning. Look at the word carefully **DIE-**t. No, that is not a typo. I just wanted to point out that the word diet starts with the word die! This perfectly makes my case for why diets are no good!

Dieting just made me angry and mean and upset because I wanted to enjoy food and eat what I wanted. I was never one to gorge on food or over indulge. I like good food and I loved eating it and depriving me of this pleasure did not seem like a good idea.

There had to be a better way to lose weight, get healthy and feel my best because this was not cutting it for me. As every day passed I was in more pain, not happy with what I had to do and was losing ground. Here is a clue to people; when it is their idea they are happy. Dieting was not my idea but one I was taught and told was the only way to go so I took it on. They were wrong with their idea and so was I.

My Story

In February of 2007 I was 336 pounds. Look on the front cover and you will see where I started my journey. Puffy face, well rounded, larger than life and baggy clothes. I started as I stated with exercise and dieting in that month and here is what went on for 4 years as I tackled this issue head on.

From 2007 until 2010 I went through a roller coaster ride. I would hit the exercise regimen and diet hard, lose about 50 pounds and then could not get out of bed and by the beginning of spring all the weight I had lost had found me once again. For four years this was a continuous cycle. It was maddening and very frustrating.

Luckily during this time period I had decided to also do a ton of research and figure out if there was a better way to losing weight and feeling better. I did all the things I described and all the while researching and testing and investigating for something better. I knew if I was struggling, so were millions of other people.

Well, after almost four years of going through this roller coaster ride of losing weight and putting it back on, I had decided that enough was enough. I needed a restart and I needed it right then and there because I was at my wits end.

I knew that I was heading towards forty and if I did not get this under control now that it may be impossible to ever get it under control. I also knew I hated the way I felt although most would never know it as I always appeared to feel good about myself and was very active and had a smile on my face most of the time.

That is what peaked my interest in trying to figure out weight loss and that was how I felt even though I was so heavy. I felt like I was sexy as hell and I never saw that picture on the front cover when I looked in the mirror. I looked in the mirror and saw awesomeness! I was the most desirable man alive in my head and the mirror showed me no different. I didn't want to lose weight because I thought I looked bad. I wanted to lose weight because I knew it was wearing me down and didn't feel great.

336 Pounds and the Lies We Tell Ourselves About Weight Loss

Right now, as you are sitting there reading this book, you are at a body weight that is either perfect for you, is an okay body weight or is no where you want to be with your body weight. Most are in the last two categories I would suspect. The place to start with and ask about your weight is this; why don't I like the body weight I am at and what would be my ideal weight?

I didn't like the way my clothes hung off of me. I hated it and to compensate for it I would buy expensive clothes and bigger clothes sizes. I was as high as a triple X at one point. That size didn't fit me but, it was comfortable and the clothes loose so that is what I cared about at the time. So as I think about my triple x comfort clothes it reminds me of the lies we tell ourselves about weight loss.

I think this is a perfect spot to talk about the lies about weight loss. I just told you I bought bigger clothes that were loose to feel better yet I felt bad because of the way my clothes looked. One of these is the truth and I want to help you to stop the crazy lies right here right now. The longer you hold on to these ideas, the longer you will hold onto the weight you currently have.

Now as I talk about the lies and give my opinions, I am going to be brutally honest. When I talk about certain aspects of weight, being fat and other aspects, I am not saying that you are not beautiful inside or that I hate people who are overweight. Remember I was one of them too but, what I am saying is what needs to be said and heard when it comes to being overweight, fat, and obese.

Here is a lie I can't stand to hear; I am happy with my weight because I am perfect the way I am. You have to throw this idea away right now because if you were happy as you are you would not be reading this book, always on a diet and having a love affair with your food. What is wrong with declaring that you are fat and you are tired of your thighs rubbing together! You have to own up to where you are at with your weight and quit lying to yourself. Happy with your weight and happy with whom you are can be two different scenarios and should be if you are going to be honest about losing weight.

Another classic is that plus size women are beautiful. Again I do not know how they might be as people but, being fat, obese and carrying extra flab around is not sexy, beautiful or otherwise. You don't have to feel worthless and you can be as beautiful as you like on the inside but, your outside is screaming for help. We were not meant to be fat as it is our food, society, mindset and thinking that has us bulging at the seams. You may be a very beautiful soul and person but, let's face the facts and that is your butt, stomach and arms are unsightly. Get yourself motivated and truthful and make those body parts what you desire. If you are happy with them as they are then that is all that matters. Close this book because you will not need what I have to offer here.

I eat for comfort is also a classic lie or excuse as well because the more you eat, the more uncomfortable you get. How can you even think you feel comfort? I know you feel guilt and stress and you are trying to find a feel good feeling but, there is no comfort involved I assure you. Your brain is tricking you into thinking you are comfortable and warm feeling. You know it and I know it that you are harming yourself with every bite.

Food is an addiction for me and I can't help it is right up there with the tops lies. First off you can help what you put in your mouth so never give up your power to anything. Second, food is great in all with moderation but, over indulging in anything is miserable and not addicting.

I have always been over weight so what is the point? I'll always be overweight! Nothing last forever and just because something has always been does not have to mean it will always be this way. You are in charge of who you are, what you are and what you want to be so take charge of you and do not give in. I know losing weight is tough and at times can be depressing but, I promise you that you can be something new and improved. Life is about transformation and second chances.

I am not fat. I am just big boned! If you are just big boned then let's sees some bones and not all of the extra padding you are carrying around. You may be big boned but ultimately you are overweight and need to lose it.

It is not my fault that I am overweight because I had a baby. I love the fact that you had a baby and put on the weight from having one but if the baby is born then it is time to shed those pounds. Lose the excuse so you will be happier. Mommies do not have to be obese or curvy just because they had a baby. I know life gets tougher with children but ultimately you do not need excuses you need results.

I can go on and on all day long with all of the lies about weight loss but, what is the point really? Here is how to sum it all up; if you are making excuses about your weight in any way then it is time to give them up and change. If you do not feel good about your weight then it is time to change. Fatty, saggy skin all dimpled and stretched out is not sexy in any way. Please be honest about that. Trying to find clothes that fit right when you are obese is not fun in any way. You want better for yourself and you deserve better.

Be honest at all times and call it what it is and that is being fat is not fun and you want to change it! No more lies, only new truths and then on to your ideal weight.

Prepare Your Mind for Food

It was one night when I was watching one of those news shows when I was watching how these two people, one man and one woman could increase their body temperature and get in freezing water and come out of it with no issues and most shockingly alive. I watched with intensity and was amazed at what I was watching and was questioning if this was real or even possible. They both had the same thing to say and that is that they used the power of their mind in order to make this happen. They actually raised their body temperature once in the water which is incredible.

I sat their thinking back to something I had done for years; I could go out into a snow storm in shorts and a jacket and would never be cold while doing this. I told myself as long as I had a jacket and my upper body was warm then I was okay. I had determined that in my mind and it made me think even deeper about other realities I had created in my mind.

I wondered if I could apply this to my body in regards to weight loss, health and fitness and personal growth. I mean it is not that farfetched even back when I realized this because I had been doing it many different ways in my life already. I knew right then and there I had something but, I wondered why more people did not realize how to utilize this incredible power. These two people were amazing and I felt like it was ground breaking.

From that point forward I was on a mission to change life for myself and when it worked, the life of others as well. I wanted to see how I could leverage this new information for my benefit and yours to help me lose weight with my mind.

So the foundation for this whole book and the How to Think You Way to Thin program is based around the power of the mind and if you are not properly utilizing the mind then this will never work for you. You must clear your mind of toxic thoughts and re-program your thinking in the way you think about food, weight and healthy living. Even if you are wheel chair bound this will work as long as your mind still works like normal then you can participate in this program.

Before I ever place food in my mouth I remove all negative thoughts about it. I am not stressed and I have no guilt. I do not focus on losing weight. I use the power of my mind to do something very powerful and ensure that my body wakes up and goes to work on burning fat. Everything I eat is fat burning food. More on this later as we journey on but, I felt it is a very important element to begin to understand.

Fat is a State of Mind

Why do I say that fat is a state of mind? Simple, when I was fat and at my heaviest, my mindset was not the best it could be. I was lazy at times, didn't care about consequences of food or alcohol and I did not have the right mindset. I was fat because of the way that I thought. I was still a good person with great qualities just not with my health and eating habits or mindset of food like I should have been.

I generally do not believe in stereotypes yet there are a few exceptions; I believe that most people who are seriously overweight have common mindsets and activities that define them. Before you get upset with me I am not here to make you feel bad or insult anyone. I am here to make sure that I bring as much as I can to your attention so you will own up to the bad decisions you are making and what it will take to get you to the best decisions you can make.

I am sure there are many people in this world with medical conditions that can explain why they are heavy. I am not here to judge but, now that you are heavy, what are you going to do about changing it? Being overweight has a tenancy to create feelings, mindsets and emotions. It tends to change your perspective and how you think about life.

If you want to change your world then my answer will always be the same; then change your mind. Don't think like a fat person, or talk like a fat person or eat like a fat person. Think thin, act thin and be thin! Yes, there is more to the program but, this is where we are going to concentrate our efforts; mindset!

To me, a true disability is when we say we can't and not because we have a disease, illness, missing limbs or a reason for how our body is in the current state that it is in. It is amazing how empowering the words are, "I can or I will." I can lose weight. I will make this happen. I can lose weight mentally. Go ahead and say these words, "I can lose the weight I want to and be healthy." How did that feel to say out loud?

Family History

Where does family history come into play with weight loss or worse with weight gain? Keep in mind I am not a doctor and I am strictly giving my opinions and observations but, my beliefs on family history in regards to weight loss or gain is that we are all individuals and there for can decide how you are going to be when it comes to your weight.

When you observe an entire family that is obese or overweight, you might think they are all bound to be that way because of genetics. If you were to eat dinner at the house and hang around for a few days you might find something different. What you might find is bad food in the house, poor eating habits, over indulging, lack of movement and poor or obese attitudes. I am not saying this holds true for all obese families and I am not trying to be mean but, I have found this to be true 95% - 98% of the time of the obese families that I have observed including my own family.

Family history is more about habits and lifestyles and less about genetic and destiny. You can end up where you want to but, if you do not break free from these habits learned from your family then you will all follow the same path. This makes complete sense I hope. You learn to eat what your family eats and think about food the way your family does unless you change it.

When I was younger we drank whole milk until I graduated high school, cooked in old grease saved on the counter and had very little vegetables. My family was not what you would call "*health nuts.*" I did most of that on my own. I never changed it until I was in high school when I was a serious athlete. How could I change something that I did not know any better? I did what my family did as it was a continuous cycle of learned behaviors.

Break the cycle and try and change up a few things at first. Look up everything you are eating and get rid of a couple of things that are really bad for you. One thing I did when I was changing habits was I switched to two percent milk and then down to one percent milk. This was a big switch for me and one that was a good thing to change. I look at vitamin D milk today and it makes me sick.

Where Does Exercise Come in?

The first thing we need to discuss about exercise is the way we look at it. When I exercise I do not call it exercise as negative connotations come to my mind right away. I call it getting movement for my body. I do it because I feel better when I am not stiff. If I feel obligated to work out and sweat I often have a bad attitude and realize this is counterproductive to my health. See I am no different than you when it comes to exercise and I realize that I have to change my mind about it. I do enjoy at times a good workout but most of the time I have other things I would rather do.

So that is what I decided to do one day; I changed the way I looked at getting exercise. I knew that as I was getting older I was less likely to do the things that I had done in my teens and twenties. All the way up to the point in my 30's I was willing to do whatever it took to stay in shape. Once I hit my mid-thirties it was an entirely different story. I no longer wanted to work out with a fury as I was in a different phase of life.

One of the things I have noticed about getting older is that the less we move the stiffer we get. The stiffer we get the less likely we are to exercise, move or feel great for that fact. Flexibility equals movement and better health.

People often ask me if I am serious that I never exercised when I lost the 105 pounds and the truth is that I exercised next to nothing until I had lost about 90 plus pounds and even then I went for long walks. I mainly did this because I could and felt like I wanted to.

I had made the mistake several times of exercising as I stated before and this time I wanted to succeed and my mind set was everything to me so I wanted nothing in my way. I did not want to break down and have my body feel like it was at a breaking point.

At some point once you start to lose a significant amount of weight I will guarantee you that you will want to get your body moving. A body in motion tends to stay in motion and nothing feels better than moving and stretching and feeling healthy. I assure you though that I am not going to teach you to work out. That is another subject in itself and I want you to focus on accessing the brain for your weight loss right now.

The secret to my weight loss comes from my mindset and my mental exercises. The by-product of my weight loss and mindset is a healthier life style which now affords me to be able to get out more and enjoy movement and walking and taking in the sites. At three hundred and thirty six pounds I needed more rest and less movement. Every step at the time was an event and although I was strong I was also very weak from all of the weight I carried.

If we position our minds in the way we should we can tackle anything we desire and I decided that I would lose this weight with my mind in the right way. I learned to exercise internally first. I visualized working out mentally just like I would physically.

You must get your body moving inside in order to make this concept work. Focus on it and have it on your mind all of the time. Visualize your machine getting cranked up and moving. Your blood is flowing at maximum capacity and your organs all functioning at the best they can. You are invincible and you have the capability to be your best. You are going to laugh at how well this way of thinking works. I visualize these things several times a day.

Next, you need to get started on cranking up your inside. Vision you running in your favorite place. Feel your organs and your muscles working at their best. Raise your hands in celebration as you are in charge of your body and the race. Do some visual crunches, push-ups and some stretching.

Now you may think that this is silly and if so I understand because for a second I did at first too but, very quickly I realized what was silly was three hundred and thirty six pounds. So I did these exercise several times a day with disciplines and the silliness quickly went away.

Several times throughout my day when I was working at my desk I would do things like flex my stomach in increments of twenty and then my buttocks in the same way. I would do leg lifts off of the floor a few inches and hold. I have a flex ball I use to work my wrists. I stretch my arms and legs even sitting at my desk.

About 10 months ago I bought a total gym and is one of the lowest impact workouts I have ever done. It is perfect for those who do not like working out. No worries as I do not kill myself on it. I like it because it fits in with the mindset I have and the mental weight loss process. If you are not interest in working out then no worries but if you want to do some kind of work out I suggest that you look into this machine.

Today I move as often as I can because I feel great! As we continue on we will work together to get you feeling great as well but, I urge you to take everything I am saying as serious as you can. I have seen it work with my own eyes. You can do this I promise you!

Before My Feet Hit the Ground Out of Bed

I do not know if you understand how important your first thoughts of the day are before you get out of bed but, I can tell you that they set your day. How they set your day is entirely up to you. Words are powerful so please choose wisely!

I used to just get up out of bed and head towards the shower. Today I have a totally different routine as before I jump out of bed and put my feet on the ground I have a whole mental routine that I go through. It is not long and it is not complicated but, it helps me to get my day going right and it sets my machine in motion (the body – more about this in chapter 3)

I lay there and get myself awake and then I tell myself to get my machine moving. Slowly it starts and gets into a good rhythm. Faster and faster it moves as I feel my body start to come alive. I focus on one thing that is very important and that is I tell my body that today is a high fat burning day and I need it to get moving on the process.

I visualize fat melting away in my body and I picture my stomach and whole body getting leaner. Once I feel that I am at full charge, I then get myself out of bed and head to the shower. While I am in the shower I pray, act as grateful as I can for the day given to me, do some stretching (warm water is good for muscles for this) and I focus in on the healing power of my brain on my body.

I know what you could be thinking after hearing some of this; does he really do this every day? Is this stuff real? How come more people do not talk about this stuff if it is real?

First off, yes I really do this every day and would not consider missing a day of doing the exercises even if I was miserably sick. Second, yes this is as real as it gets and you will find out quick it works. Third, this takes a lot of discipline and faith. It is just not main stream (yet) and has not been brought to light as it should. That is why I am writing this book because I think it is too big of a discovery to be kept a secret.

Chapter 2 –Dissatisfaction

Instead of giving myself reasons why I can't, I give myself reasons why I can.~ **Unknown Author**

I avoided taking pictures as I never liked the way I looked in them for quite a few years. I never could put my finger on why but, I just didn't like the way I looked. You would have thought a picture of me would have done the trick but, it didn't dawn on me as I thought I was just not photogenic at times. After several diets and exercise programs failures what really drove me to dissatisfaction was a trip to the mall.

I love good clothes and everything I came across one day was the most frustrating thing I had been through. I was too big for regular clothes and too small for the big and tall clothes. I mean is this really my life? I was at my wits end and needed to do something about it.

I was not happy either the way my clothes hung off me. It was like wearing drapes at times as I went bigger and bigger with my clothes so they would hang off of me and not cling to me. All I wanted was to be cool and comfortable.

I would often go places and need to rest a lot. I would sweat on a cool winter day and become out of breath walking up stairs. I hate to sweat and I was doing more and more of it. I never really hated who I was as a person but, I hated who I had become as a body. There was a skinny and healthier me in there somewhere but, it was hard to see it with all of the body that had formed around my bones.

After going through so many emotions, diets and more, I had finally become dissatisfied enough to make drastic changes. When you are satisfied you will not change things. When you have finally had enough and the will and desire are there to do something then magical things can occur. I had finally reached that point in my life where I was going to make a change.

I do not believe that you have to hit rock bottom in order to make drastic changes. I just believe that you have to be at a point where you will no longer accept something that has been happening in your life. You have to decide you want something better and you have to decide to make the changes.

Once I had decided that I wanted to lose this weight and make drastic change I went through several stages along the way. The stage I needed to finally arrive at was the one I needed to finally get to where I wanted. That stage was called my new reality. That stage where you make it a part of your everyday life and there is no other option. It is where I was resolved to make it a part of who I was with no turning back.

I wanted to be the best me and was not going to settle until I made this my new reality. I had the mindset and I had the passion but, what I needed was the means to get there in a healthy way.

Negative and Harmful Thoughts

Lying about your weight is as bad as having poor internal conversations and negative thoughts. All of these have a huge impact on you and your thoughts and mindset as well as your health. Negative and harmful thoughts will not help you lose weight. Your thoughts are so powerful and if you allow your thoughts to slip to a negative state then your health will suffer. There is a powerful balance that must take place in your mind about whom you are and where you want to be and having the right attitude is paramount to losing weight mentally.

Before I took off the weight, I had a mentality of a guy who could do anything and seemed like I had the world wired. What I had not realized yet was that when it came to food I did not have it wired right in my mind. The food was in control, bad thoughts and stress and looking at my gut did not help either. Everything to do with food and my weight literally stressed me out and because of it I had a bad attitude.

To make matters worse I felt like I was the bomb. I acted like the sexiest man alive and the only thing sexy about me was my confidence because my body was not it for sure. I was built very strong which was good but, I also had a lot of body fat by way of poor mental choices and life style decisions.

At times during this book and my program you may get confused by some of what I say but, I assure you that once we are done you will understand what I am laying out for you. If there is any confusion at this point then you will have clarity real soon. For clarification purposes to this point we must know that bad thoughts equal bad weight and health. I like to keep it simple and this one is as simple as it gets in my book.

You will never catch me saying or insinuating that we have to be all positive in order to achieve what we desire. I do not believe that if we are just positive in life we will achieve whatever we want. However it is important to have a positive attitude at times and more importantly if you harbor negative thoughts and bad attitudes then you are asking for nothing but hard times and bad health.

The better my attitude was, the better thoughts I had and the better my outlook, the more weight I lost. Along the way I had a little weight put back on and guess what was going on in my life; stress, bad thoughts and crappy ideas and as soon as I removed that from the equation I lost the weight again and more and have kept it off since.

What is happening in your life right now? Are you stressed? What do your internal conversations sound like? Do you keep your thoughts positive and real?

Binge Eating – Emotions

I grew up in a family with a few alcoholics involved in our life and I learned something very powerful not only about alcoholics but, about life and what we call binge eaters as well; after you drink yourself into oblivion the problems you are trying to avoid will still be there when you sober up. The same holds true with binge eating and your problems and worries.

This is not a sub-chapter on binge eating or comfort eating but, really an explanation of why you have to remove the problem from the equation. Comfort foods binge eating or depression eating all comes with emotions. Eating for any kind of comfort is debilitating and wrong for you. We need to correct whatever takes you to this state of eating first if you want to succeed in losing the weight you want to.

The food we eat send signals to our brains because of two things ultimately; the first is in response to what is in the food such as sugars, carbs, etc. The second type of signal sent to our brain and in my opinion the most important one is the signal we send because of how we feel while we are eating. We send joy, guilt, stress, laughter, satisfaction, happiness, feelings of bonding, etc. We send those signals because that is what we decided pasta night is on Thursdays or Christmas dinner every year.

It is extremely important that we take responsibility for our thoughts and food signals we send to the brain because they will occur either consciously or sub-consciously. Meaning either you will be at the controls or your mind will be on auto-pilot. I'd rather make my own decisions as I go and control the responses.

If you get stressed and then go and hide in a bowl of ice crème and you continue to repeat this process then you know what will happen because life will always have stress events as they will not go away. What you have control over is the events you tie to your stress and eating should never be one of them!

When I stress I tend to stop what I am doing and refocus myself. I tend to get some movement and think quietly. I tend to reflect and examine my actions. I do not let food in or alcohol or any other kind of distraction until I solve the problem. I hate it when I read Facebook and someone has a problem and their answer is getting drunk or needing a beer. Even if they are kidding (generally they are not) I understand the long term effects from this mentality.

Focus on the solution first and double layer chocolate cake is not the solution. Ben and Jerry's Ice Cream has never had a registered therapist on payroll as far as I know. The solution is where you can remove the binge eating habits you acquired. More than likely if you are a binge eater you learned it from a family member. They probably never told you how to do it, you just watched, observed and then started doing it. If you have kids or are getting ready to, then they are probably going to do the same thing unless you change it now.

My binge eating now is so much different than before. I eat for raw strength, weight loss or fuel. I do not eat ever because I have to eat or because I am stressed. I also try and never eat when I am exhausted either. Have you ever noticed that when you are so tired and starved that you eat sugary foods? You tell yourself you are tired and need something to give you energy or a pick you up now feeling. Try and eat when you are not tired and watch how much less you will have the desire to eat.

Eating poorly really is about living poorly mentally. You have to want to turn your body into a thriving machine that eats up nutrients and provides fuel. You have to want to turn on the sunshine inside of you and keep it on twenty four hours a day. You have to want to be a peak performer no matter what you do for a living. My system is about concentrating on your body and freeing your mind so that it does not release toxins into the body!

Where we do not want to comfort eat or binge eat, we also do not want to skip meals either because by doing this your body flips out. It knows are trying to starve it so it stores fat instead while you are doing this in order to protect it. Essentially you can put on wait while living in misery of not eating. That is crazy but true so we need to fuel our body on a regular basis in small increments.

My mom had it right when she used to say most things in moderation are good for you. This holds very true for food because moderation is what the body can handle. You never want to feed yourself too much of anything or starve the body of everything. Feed your machine the proper way and without the emotional roller coaster.

The Problems with Alcohol

Where do we start with the problems of alcohol! There are many things we can talk about when it comes to alcohol but that is another lesson for another time. My focus for this book is weight loss and mental health. The problems with alcohol when it comes to losing weight are where we will start and then you will decide if you should drink on a regular basis or even casually.

One of the biggest problems I know about alcohol when it comes to your body is that when you take in alcohol your body gives it first priority when it comes to digestion. In reality if you drink alcohol and eat finger foods, appetizers or anything else, the body deals with the alcohol first and stores the rest as fat to may be dealt with later. This should be a big eye opener for you and give you a clue why you put on weight when you drink.

Also, alcohol equals sugar and could really be added to my 50 names for sugar. I do not like the name beer belly but I do like the name sugar belly. Sounds nicer and gives a better visual to me. Bottom line is alcohol is sugar to your belly and you do not need that.

When you drink I am sure you do other unhealthy things like skip water intake, eat out on a lot of unhealthy foods and possible other undesirable activities. I know my wife and I loved to throw parties when we lived in Seattle and we loved having yummy food and making sure everyone was having a great time. We brought out the entire smiley foods to the party. You know what I mean, sugary foods, chips, snacks, fatty meats and more. The foods that make you smile. Alcohol gets you fired up and the appetite kicks in.

That should give you some pretty good insights why you might want to avoid alcohol while you are trying to lose weight. I do not want to bum you out or make you feel stressed but you need to understand what is fighting against you in your weight loss battle.

Smart Weight Loss

I believe one of the smartest things I did during my weight loss journey was to determine what smart weight loss really was. When I first started on the journey, I had ideas of dropping thirty pounds at a time like I was slicing off bread and every time I did this I put it back on. In chapter 3 you will learn about my eating habits and you will discover quickly that it went along with my weight loss goals once I finally realized responsible weight loss.

The fact of the matter is that you put on weight the same way I did; once by once and pound by pound. If you are going to identify what responsible weight loss is then you must recognize how you put it on.

My goals for losing the weight were very simple once I realized how I put it on. I wanted to lose a pound a week and no more. I know that may sound strange especially when you are carrying around over a hundred pounds of fat sack but, I learned something very powerful along the way. Natural will always be natural and when it is not natural then it can harm you greatly. In other words there is no magic and Mother Nature always works best! Work within the system of your body and do not fight or work against it.

So on my way I went focusing on losing a pound a week. I had it in my brain all day every day and when you read on and learn some of the small activities I did, you will begin to see how all of this stuff starts to tie together. There is no one piece to this puzzle you can do and skip the rest. I am giving you a complete system and you have to use it that way as a whole.

I am telling you the truth when I say you do not have to diet or exercise. You will have to get yourself moving and you will have to put goodness into your body as well as you will have to focus on what you want but, nothing crazy or painful!

This one strategy alone has some great power to it as if you will focus in on what you want in the way of weight loss or really anything and you allow yourself to think about it morning, noon and night, then you will begin to see how it will start to take shape. Focus on what you want in life instead of focusing on what you do not want in your life. I do not want to be fat will surely make you fat. I want to lose a pound a week and get skinny is affirming to your mind.

Smart weight loss is taking weight off the same way that you put it on and with the proper focus you can chip away at the weight naturally and healthy. I wanted a pound a week but you might be fine with a half of a pound a week depending on your size and goals.

Doing Little Things for Big Results

One of the hardest things when you want to lose weight is that everything seems so big to take on and not just the expanding mid-section you are carrying. Everything you think about doing seems like a daunting task and so before you get started you have already quit. Like everything in this book mindset and attitude determines everything and all along your weight loss journey you will need to adjust both your attitude and your mindset to take advantage of better thoughts and ideas.

At the peak of my weight gain, I was lethargic and my movement was at an all-time low. To think about going out for a jog when I was my heaviest was a horrible idea to throw at me and I would rather go and hit my head against the wall until I passed out. So going on a big exercise program was out for me. As you already know I tried that any ways and it about crippled me.

I love food and enjoy food (or at least I did a lot) and so going on a diet of broccoli and rice cakes was a slow and certain death for me. I'd rather choke to death on hot dogs and coca cola before I went on a diet so that was out of the equation for me too. One of my favorite jokes comes from a comedian who calls himself fluffy. What fluffy says is that he would rather eat a taco today knowing that he could die tomorrow and that is the way I felt about my food.

Here is what I knew to be true though once I had decided I was serious; I needed little bits and pieces of this stuff if I wanted to live healthier and longer and I knew that good health was about movement and foods that maximized my body's efficiency.

The idea I had was that I did not need to do big things or exercises or diets that were hard on my body but, what I needed to do was a little something every once in a while which was more than I was currently doing at the time. I'd take a short, easy stroll to the end of the street or go work in my garden or make a planter box. I just needed movement!

I needed more vegetables so I would eat a little of this or that and give myself the best chance at all of the nutrition I could get. I took supplements and vitamins and drank more water all the while I was eating the foods I still wanted. Foods and drinks are not the main problem in your life; it's the way you think about them, ignore them, abuse them and stop doing the little things that you should be doing.

If you are desk bound, wheel chair bound or bed bound, there is something you can be doing to get yourself moving and in better shape. At the very worst you have your mind and because of that you have every chance in the world to be better.

Do not stress depending on your situation because there is always hope and you are never permanently anything. You dictate your future and the only thing holding you back is you. You have the chance to take this weight off, get moving and feel great! The world has so much to offer and you need to get to where you can enjoy a 100% of it.

How Did You Get Here to Begin With?

We all have reasons why we end up where we end up in life. Everyone and I mean everyone has a story and I am certain that you are no different than the rest. I also know that you have every reason for being thirty pounds overweight or maybe even a whole lot more. Let me ask you a question, "does it really matter?"

If you believe that you have a great reason for being overweight do these reasons help you with feeling better about your weight? Do you sweat less, breathe lighter and do your clothes fit better? You see, having a reason really does nothing for you including helping your self-esteem. What you need is to have a reason to lose the weight and eliminate the reasons or excuses.

Like you, I have had plenty of reasons to put on the weight and because of those reasons I had created plenty of poor behaviors. Behaviors that went along with the reasons to allow me to eat in a certain way or think in a certain way and this are what really caught my attention with mental weight loss because of the mental weight gain that happened. Think about that idea and let it sink in. I put on weight with poor mental thoughts so why could I not take it off with good mental thoughts?

So I determined that I had to go to work and fix or replace the behaviors and ideas that I had created with my reasons. Get rid of the baggage and start fresh for the calmer your mind is the better it will perform. Baggage or things we hold onto mentally always have repercussions. There is no such thing as good baggage.

If you will take the time to analyze and reflect, I promise you that you will start seeing what I did when I started on my journey. I had so many reasons in my life for being fat which ranged from being too busy to eat right to deserving it to stress and many more reasons. I knew they were just excuses but, they delivered momentary comfort along with long term pain.

In order to become successful, we always need to understand where we are starting from. Do you know how you got to where you are at right now? Do you know where you want to go? If you know the beginning and the ending but don't know how to make the journey, then this book will be your guide. For now make sure you are clear on the pathway here so you can find the pathway back to where you want to be.

Top Ways to Sabotage Yourself

I think that it is important to understand some of the ways that people often sabotage themselves when they are trying to lose weight and get healthy. I do not want to be negative but, we should understand some of the lies, the hurdles and setbacks to a healthier you!

Tell no lies! Whatever the truth is in your life let it ring through and do not create a new story. The more truthful you are with yourself, the more truthful your life will be as a whole. Nothing will sabotage your weight loss quicker than living a bunch of untruths so let go of all those feelings that you have tied to situations and live free from self lies.

Eating for comfort is a no-no. If you need comfort in a time of stress then it is time to change where you get the comfort from. Find comfort in a book, watching a movie or talking to a friend but, eliminate food from the equation. Comfort food will make you fat and obese in no time so change this habit right now. You decided food was comforting and you can decide that something else is more comforting.

People give up before they start to lose weight because it is too hard. I would imagine that 95% of the people who try to lose weight give up within two weeks to a month because of the frustration of wanting to lose weight now. If you quit then you will never hit your goals. If you quit then you will never get to the weight that makes you feel your best.

Feeling guilty over your weight and food intake and anything else will sabotage your success quick. You might think that feeling guilty would keep you honest but, guilt often has the opposite effect as it will crush you and leave you feeling exhausted. You must learn to live guilt free no matter what is happening. Everything I eat now has no guilt tied to it as I smile every fork of food I eat.

I am not going to lie to you as weight loss is hard to a certain degree and it will take some time. I learned right away to have some patience in the matter of losing weight. Not a lot of patience because successful people are impatient but, to be real I had to not rush the experience so I would not get frustrated and want to quit. I knew in my heart I was going to lose weight and did not waver for the most part. You should be confident in your journey as well. Once the weight starts coming off do not let up and do not lose your focus. Your number one job is to remain focused and keep that brain working on burning fat.

Lose Weight for the Right Reasons

What are your reasons for losing weight? Are you tired of being called fat? Do you worry about what people think? Does your spouse want you to lose weight? I know it sounds like common sense but, you must lose weight for the right reasons and losing weight so someone will like you or look at you is not the right reason.

Most people often fail not only at weight loss as well as many other goals because they are not properly motivated.

Being properly motivated is not a fake superficial feeling. Being properly motivated is having the proper understanding of exactly what you want, focusing on what you want and being enthusiastic about the process to get there. If your reasons for losing weight are not serious enough or filled with enough consequences then you will surely not push through and lose the weight that you need to. If you are just excited at the thought of losing a few dress sizes but not the actual journey then it is more than likely going to fade quickly.

If you are overweight right now that is reason enough but, it is too broad or general of an idea. You need to laser down and focus in on the finite reasons you MUST lose weight. For instance; I want to lose weight is too general but I want to lose weight so I can play with my kids outside without breathing heavy and feeling is specific.

My reasons were that my clothes did not feel well, my health was at risk, I have a family that needs me and my body was aching. My family extended family has died way too early and I wanted to change that. I understood the side effects of obesity and I wanted to avoid the death sentence that it carried.

Losing weight for the right reasons may seem a bit confusing but, really it is very easy to understand. For instance, if my wife tells me I have to lose weight then I feel stressed and I reject the idea even though I love her and want to make her happy. If on my own I want to lose weight and one of my motivations is I want to be healthy for my wife and kids then I am okay with the idea. There is no stress in the second idea, just motivation and although it seems like the same thing I promise you it is very different. I decide my fate and destiny and I create my own happiness and I lose the weight I want for the reasons I create.

Magazines and the media today have created images of what you should look like and the weight you should be at. They influence people's minds on how to dress and how to feel but, the truth of the matter is that you should be determining all of that stuff and not someone sitting in New York City. That life is not necessarily yours if that is not what you are looking for.

This type of marketing is designed to stress you out and influence you the way the media wants you to go. Take away the stress and just gather ideas and then formulate what you desire. When you decide what you want and how things will be then you will be happier.

Avoid peer pressure of any kind as well because what is needed is an authentic you. It is always okay to get ideas by looking at other people but, they are ideas and not something that should become a stress point. Make sure that you always living your own life and design your own body and ideal weight. Believe it or not some people are not meant to be ninety five pounds.

How is that Diet Working For You?

Why do you think that diets do not work? I believe that starting a diet is like taking a Saint Bernard and stuffing it through the cat door. Some things just do not fit. A diet is like that forced situation and trying to push you into a diet spells failure right from the start.

Let's be honest and talk about what goes on in a diet situation. You are supposed to stick to foods that are healthy. The problem I believe with the so called "healthy" food is it often is not really healthy and usually tastes blah and boring to us. There is no creamy filling in the middle that squirts out or sprinkles on top. How are you supposed to be happy when you are eating things that make you unhappy?

What I find in this "healthy" food is that you will try and buy foods that say no fat all to find out they are loaded in sugar or sodium. You might lose a pound but, in the mean time you have to be put on blood pressure medicine.

The healthy alternatives are expensive to purchase and they can zap a budget real quick. What you suddenly begin to do is conserve on eating the food so it will last. Your mood is starting to take you to a place called unhappy times because this is changing and lessoning your life style. Next time you go shopping you substitute a few things to make things last longer and five shopping trips later you barely have a carrot in your shopping cart.

Diet; is there any coincidence that there is the word "die" in diet? Okay I know I am messing around but, if you are like me I would rather die than diet as it is a miserable experience. There are so many reasons that diets do not work but, the main reason is that they are forced and a major disruption to your life.

No one really goes on a diet because they want to. They diet because they have to and that is where the rub comes in. As a human being we resist pressure no matter where it comes from and a diet is pressure. You are doomed to resist it because of the un-natural process that it takes you through. Do not get me wrong in what I am saying because we should eat as healthy as we can. I know you understand what I am saying because you are not a fan of dieting either.

So how is that diet working for you? How much goodness has a diet every delivered to your life? Have you ever had a successful diet that worked and helped you to keep the weight off? I am sure there are a few who would say yes and I would not get into any kind of debate with them but, what I would say is that diets start and have to be stayed on in order to be successful long term. Dieting is how you lost the weight and have kept the weight and because of that you are dependent on the diet.

In my opinion the only successful diet is one that you don't have to be dependent on. That is why dieting does not work because there are none that this is possible with.

Become the Body Type You See

It is easy to see the body that you are right now but, do you clearly see the body type that you want to become? If you cannot see the body that you want to look like in your mind then you will always struggle to reach a destination that will make you happy! You must first vision it and then focus on it and then make it happen.

If you have made it this far in the book and you are not yet understanding my mindset training for weight loss then let me help make it extremely clear; If you cannot clear your mind of the bad and focus on what you want with a clear vision and a positive charge then nothing else you do will matter much. Mental weight loss is about brain power. It is about your ability to create a vision in your mind that you will create in real life.

The key to achieving anything great in life is the ability to see things that have not yet arrived in your life. Success comes from the brain and your thoughts and your ability to vision. Success also comes from eliminating the negative thoughts you possess. Removing the self-doubt and the debilitating thoughts you are holding on to. Am I starting to make it clear yet?

Let me take it one step further in the hopes I can pound home the ideas that are going to help you finally lose weight. I will bet that you are where you are at with your weight because of life's stress and pressure, the fact that you are getting older is playing in as a factor and the fact that you can't see another position you could be in with your weight except to keep getting heavier. Therefore, where you are is exactly where you have put yourself. If I am not dead on I bet that I am close if you are honest about it.

You must take responsibility both for Weight gain and weight loss and the responsibility is critical. Every aspect to weight loss and weight gain is and was at your hands and once you take responsibility for that then you can own up to it and make your new reality happen.

** Action Item**

Spend 5 minutes, close your eyes, sit in a quiet place and visualize what your new body will look like in the near future. See every aspect from your thighs to your stomach, ankles and arms. Smile the whole time while you are visualizing as you will feel something very powerful happen.

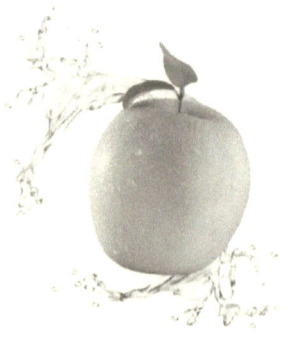

Chapter 3 – Getting Your Machine (Body) Working

Rule your mind or it will rule you. ~**Horace**

I came up with the idea of "the Machine" because I needed a way for my mind to focus on something else besides my body as well as a way to help teach other people how to do the same thing. I wanted to take the focus off of a frail and overweight body and put it on something that is strong, built tough and able to handle maximum power. That is why my body is not a body I have to work on but is a machine I maintain. It is massive and strong and needs to be maintained properly and is run by a computer that I control. This idea is not about fooling or lying to you. This idea is about creating a vision and a focus for you. Get the image of the machine in your mind. This machine is stories tall, has missile defense systems, is loud, powerful, has complexity to it but, is also simple in the fact that it needs fuel, and oil and maintenance and power.

I cannot fully describe the vision of the machine in my head because it is pretty wild and I really want you to create your own vision. You need to create your machine piece by piece and build it in the location that you love. Doesn't matter if it is possible just make it a reality! Once you have the picture of your machine in your mind then you must go to work focusing on it.

People that I know who are overweight and tend to go on multiple diets always focus on their body, their belly, their pants their face and all the while missing out on their mind! If you focus too much on your body then you will miss the focus of your mind. If you take control of the mind to cooperate then the body will follow.

What do you think about every day? When you are trying to lose weight what are you thinking about? Do you think about food all day? Do you focus on the fact that you are overweight? Do you obsess about the one pound you lost from last week or the two pounds that you put on this week? Are you hungry all the time and have that growl in your stomach? You see, if you do not have the right focus and you keep on thinking about these non-sense things, then weight loss is going to be incredibly difficult.

Back to the machine idea and why it is going to help you get what you want; because it works is. This focus takes away all of those wrong ideas and thoughts. The machine focus is about removing vulnerability and weakness from your daily routine and your life time struggles. By focusing on your machine you give yourself the strength that you need to go to work.

Put the next piece of the puzzle together and vision your new body called "the machine" and discover how I lost 105 pounds with mental weight loss.

My Eating Patterns

My eating habits became a great source of change in my health and it has greatly impacted how my body deals with food. Before I discuss this idea I want to describe something for you and I want you to tell me if it sounds familiar to you at all.

When I was Three hundred and thirty six pounds, I loved to eat the best food. It was the victors of my spoils as I would eat 12-16 ounce steaks, mashed potatoes and salad, plenty of drink and maybe even dessert. Then as I pushed away from the table that feeling kicked in; I had that all too familiar bloated feeling.

Now I know it may sound like I ate a lot of food but, truth be told sometimes yes I would but, most of the time I didn't. The facts are that having three big meals a day is too much food for the body to digest at one sitting. How about you? Have you ever felt bloated or stuffed? Of course you have as we all go through this common experience regularly.

The problem is that when you eat three big meals a day your body has to work really hard to digest that food and then certain foods just don't mix well in your digestion system or stomach. What I did was change the way I took in food. I mean I could not handle that feeling any longer and I was ready to lose the spare tire I had gained.

If you and I were to eat the same amount of food and drink in a day and you decided you would eat your meals three times a day while I would eat eight times a day, we would see something very interesting happen. What we would learn is that I can eat the same amount of food and drink and I would lose weight, while you will put on weight or maintain the weight. The reason is very simple; less food at a time is easier to digest and it fuels the body more efficiently and keeps the body from any major crashes. This type of eating is called "grazing" and is so good for your body in my opinion.

I really didn't change the food I ate a whole lot. What I did change was how often I ate. I would eat almost hourly some days and my body loved it! Why diet when your body is happy, running at high octane and burning calories just from eating!

Your machine loves to take in fuel and burn it efficiently and the strain on the motor is next to none when it is done the way I am explaining to you. Next time you sit down to eat and have that full plate of food, look at it and imagine it going into your stomach the size of your fist. Look at all of that mass going in your system at once and having to be digested. The body will store fat if it can't process all of it at one sitting.

When I first started breaking down my three meals into 8-10 meals a day it was a bit exhausting. I had never eaten my meals this way and planning them seemed a bit tough. Doing this method was something I was determined to do as it made so much sense. Then I stopped planning as much what I was going to eat unless I was going to be out. I ate as often as I could, little bits at a time. I still ate what I wanted and I still ate as much food initially. The biggest difference is I just spread it throughout the day instead.

After a week or so I started to get the hang of it and once again stopped stressing over it. I reminded myself to eat about every hour and half or so. My goal was to not feel hungry, let my blood sugar not get low and not feel that bloating in my gut. I started to enjoy the way I felt two weeks into it. I mean really enjoy it and was feeling great about what was happening with the experience.

Then something started to happen to my body a couple of weeks into this new way of eating; I started to get hungry again and I did not understand why. Today I understand it as I was burning my fuel at maximum capacity and my engine was revving. My machine craved the fuel in a good way and my stomach was shrinking and my metabolism was speeding up quickly.

I had not experienced this since college when I was an athlete. I was often hungry then and I ate more during that time as well as I needed the fuel. I never paid attention to it before but, I was now for sure.

Diets may not work well for you and that is fine especially if you will eat your meals like I did. In a short time you will see better results much quicker because you will stop stressing out your body and digestive system. You can do this even if you are wheel chair bound because you can speed up your metabolism and teach your body how to burn the fat and fuel more efficiently.

How Stress Plays a Role in Weight Gain

Do you understand how stress plays a role in weight gain? I am not doctor or medical researcher but, I can tell you what I know about me and my body and what I have observed in other people.

When I am stressed out I do not think clearly and my body feels stretched out like a rubber band that will not go back to shape. I want relief and I want comfort and I demand it as quickly as possible. The biggest thing about feeling stressed is the feeling of being smothered. Like the walls are closing in on me or a blanket is being pulled down on me.

I have observed this in other people as well and can see how they feel visibly. Without words you can see the reaction of people and what their body language is saying about their state. Their face becomes almost pale looking and without great expression. A cold like, ghostly look over takes their face.

If you are ever going to lose weight then you must work on removing stress and the destruction of what it brings to your life. You must realize that you are heavy on the outside because you feel heavy on the inside from life's stress and pressure and so my prayer for you is that you will learn to strip the layers of burden placed on you by you and other people and that you will lose stress weight in order to remove body weight.

When I was at my heaviest I seemed so cool, calm and collected and part of me was but, slowly but surely I was stressing out about my weight, my business, my life, my family. The more I stressed, the more I put on weight. I worked out, I focused on the right mental attitude with business and personal growth but, I always seemed to skip my health and weight.

Now at my skinniest weight in years I stress the least amount of time than I ever have. Nothing really is less stressful in my life today except I chose not give into the feelings of being stressed on a regular basis. I realize that there is good stress and there is bad stress and I steer clear of the bad as much as possible. It is merely impossible to remove all bad stress but it is possible to eliminate 90% of it from your thoughts, hearts and minds.

Seems like common sense right? Stress causes harm and if you want to live better then you need to reduce or eliminate it. The facts are this is a big struggle for most people. Stress piles on daily like dirty laundry and they struggle to remove a little of it but more piles on.

So what is the answer to stress so you can lose weight much easier? For every person you are going to have to find what works for you but, for me it is about not reacting too quick or too slow. I deal with issues head on and make sure I am being smart about what I am doing. When I mess up, I fix it. I tell it like it is even if it is not popular so I do not have to remember a lie or tippy toe around a subject.

I do not obsess over my weight or food. I laugh often and make jokes when appropriate. I work hard not to put myself in stressful situations. I am okay with failure and learn from my mistakes. I have someone I love very much as well as I love my children and my dogs and play with them when I can. All of this helps to eliminate stress in my life.

I do my best to always live within my means and not over extend myself financially. I have goals I am always working towards making sure I never obsess too much over things I want. Not stressing is about keeping life into perspective. I remove regret as much as possible as well because I observed that regret creates tension and stress in me.

Stress leads to relief and comfort and in my march towards losing 105 pounds I realized that I had a lot of stress and was constantly seeking comfort. It was not easy to lose weight let alone some of the really cool things I wanted to do because I was stressed all the time. I had to tap into my brain power and eliminate what I perceived to be pending doom and gloom. Just like the way I put on weight, I put on stress and that is one situation at a time, one thought at a time and one event at a time. To remove it I had to go about it the same way.

Incremental Change

Everything changes in this world and most of the time, if not all of the time it happens by what I call incremental change. I lost 105 pounds ounce by ounce and pound by pound because that made the most sense to me. It made sense because that is exactly how I gained it.

Everything that is built or grown is done so incrementally. A skyscraper is built a piece at a time, a pumpkin is produced off of a plant that grows incrementally and the fat on your belly was put on incrementally. It is the law of the land of how things are grown or built.

Magic would have you believe that things appear and disappear instantly. This is not true in the real world where they happen gradually. You have to come to grips with reality about how you gained the weight and how you are going to remove it. I am so glad that you realized you are overweight and that you must lose the extra baggage but, this does not mean it will come off at the speed of light and getting frustrated about it is not going to change it. Step one is to realize, step two is visualize and step three is take action.

If you want to be impatient with your weight loss then the only things you can do is exercise more and have a better attitude. You could also try the fast food action (sorry no pun intended) and have liposuction, or lap band or something like that I suppose but, if you ask me it is too dangerous, unhealthy and not a very good method as there are complications and side effects.

The other incremental change that needs to take place is the changing of your thinking and food thoughts. You will change these one at a time just like you collected them.

The Power of Water

I have water next to my bad at night for two reasons; one is I keep hydrated during the night and first thing in the morning I drink a glass to get me going. Water is powerful and it is my friend and partner in my mental weight loss.

If you tell people they need to drink more water they will say that they know that but so few people really drink the daily amount they should. In fact, most people are probably under hydrated often.

 Water is paramount for skin elasticity, proper hydration and digestion just to name a few. Water makes you feel better and helps your body to process food and waste and keep your kidneys functioning properly. Water is not some magic potion but, it is a great tool to help you with losing weight.

The type of water you drink is important as too much of anything that is not pure is harmful and can create disease in your body. There are many things that you can do today such as water filters and specialty water systems that neutralize the water and eliminate the impurities and fluoride.

Try increasing your water both first thing in the morning and late in the day and then observe the effect that it has on your body. Water is your friend and has many health benefits.

I went to Target and bought two thirty two ounce Nalgene Bottles (BPA free) and I fill them up through my filter in the fridge and I keep them in the fridge. Whenever I want to have clean, filtered water, cold and ready to go they are ready for me.

I have slowed way down buying bottled water for the most part as I learned the bottles have bad chemicals in them and they are a problem in the landfill. Water filters and Nalgene bottles are what we mostly use in our house. If I buy bottled water I buy Dasani as they are primarily made from plants.

Increasing your water intake is one way to get your body in the right direction for weight loss and by the way in case you are a diet soda drinker, these drinks have proven to cause all kinds of health issues especially if they contain alternate sugars and aspartame.

Drink water and quit fooling yourself as most of you drink diet soda out of guilt because you are over indulging on food or you think it is helping you in some healthy way. You are saving no calories or health by drink diet.

Set Your Goals and Focus

When I teach leadership to aspiring leaders, executives and sales people, I teach how to properly set goals and then I teach them how to stick up for the goals they set. Anyone can set goals but, the trick is to be accountable for them and make sure that you are going to stand behind them.

Goals without actions are just ideas and nothing more. What goals do you have for your weight loss? How much weight do you want to lose? What sizes do you want to get to for your clothes? What is your ideal weight you want to achieve?

It is extremely important to set your sights on the goals you want and with conviction. In high school in 12th grade I was 6"3" and 191 pounds and to be honest that was a bit on the thin side for me so I decided that my goal was to be two hundred pounds as that is what I visualized for me.

Anything accomplished beyond that was just icing on the cake (yes I said cake ha ha) I wanted to wear a size thirty four in pants and extra-large shirt. A large would be great but, it was ninth grade the last time I saw that size because I have broad shoulders and a big frame.

I made my goals specific and exact and not general. Too many people set general goals and do not clearly define what it is they exactly want. When you do this you end up with whatever you end up with. Be exact and ask for what you desire of yourself and the universe. Put your wants out there and focus on them and you will receive them.

How do you set goals? Do you just kind of wish for things? Do you hope that you might get some of what you want? Stop doing this to yourself and start demanding what you want. I believe that successful people are impatient and demand a lot for a reason. They understand waiting and wishing will never do them any good.

When I set goals I take everything about them serious otherwise I do not set a goal. There are no such things as having a goal you "kind of do." That is just a dream in my opinion. True goals are going to happen and losing a hundred pounds was going to happen and accomplishing it with my mind was going to happen.

You must really understand how you are going to lose weight with your mind. It is an everyday, sometime minute by minute mental game where you have conversations with yourself and make it clear what is going to happen. You must come up with the goals and then you must demand that your mind takes on what is going to happen with constant re-enforcement.

Be strong, become disciplined and ensure that you will not back down. I never backed down on what I wanted and today I am still doing it. I demand what is going on and I enforce it every day.

The reason a lot of people fail at obtaining their goals is because as the journey unfolds it gets harder and harder to hit your goal. As soon as difficult times hit then most give up and go back to comfort in their life because goals take you out of your comfort zone. Goals are tough by design so do not let tough be a reason to quit because if you can reach your goals easily then you do not have real goals. Make sure you stretch yourself far past the set boundaries.

Weight loss seems so tough because so many struggled with it and it is been well publicized. Companies sell all kinds of weight loss products and the best way these companies have figured out how to sell lots of their products is by helping you feel frustrated, helpless and like it is impossible until they introduce their miracle products.

No matter what you think to this point about the difficulty of weight loss and how hard you have tried, you can and will lose the weight you desire. You will hit your goals and you will not give up when it gets tough. The victory is yours as soon as you will declare that you will make it happen for you and your life no matter what.

Why I Cried at Macys

I was living very well and had built up some businesses like I had only dreamed of. We were living in a nice house, we had nice cars and it would seem like the world was mine. All of that was very true with two major disclaimers. The first was the passing of my mother and the second was how heavy I had risen to.

When I was in high school and college I wore a 34 in pants and a large in shirts and one day I was shopping at Macys and I was so frustrated. Everything I liked did not come in forty four waists or three XL. I could wear a two XL but that size was snug at times. I searched and searched and could not buy what I wanted. I was at a point in my life I could buy pretty much what I wanted especially with clothes and yet my money was no good. I could only buy clothes I liked but could not wear.

After an hour of looking throughout the whole store I had to find a restroom and once inside of there I just started to cry. I was not a big crier but, was not afraid to do so. Now you might think I was crying because I could not buy the clothes I wanted but, I was actually crying for another reason.

I was standing in that bathroom in Macys crying because the reality had hit me just how big I had become and was actually embarrassed for the first time ever of my weight. I had never been embarrassed before about my weight. I also had always possessed an attitude that I was good looking and sexy as hell but not on that day.

That day I was crying in the bathroom at Macys feeling sad because I had let myself get that heavy. This was not me and who I was about and I decided I must do something about it.

I will never forget that day in Macy's because it struck a chord in me so deep that every time I put on clothes I remember that day clearly. I am not sensitive and I am pretty sound as a person but that day was entirely different for me.

Inspiring others is Health Food

All along the way on your weight loss journey you will need several things to help you and inspire you. One of the things that is very powerful for both you and other people is when you start losing weight and feeling great. This is not only an inspiration but, helps others to feel that they can do something for themselves as well. Inspiring others is what I like to call mental health food because they will make you feel great and that will fuel your body and spirit.

When you decide to finally shed that weight and get your mind straight then others will start to feel that energy radiate from your energy and spirit. People will begin to be inspired by what you are doing and accomplishing.

When other people see how committed you are to your goals then they will support you and say all kinds of positive things and although this is superficial in nature as motivation goes, it is exactly what the doctor would order for you.

What hopefully will happen is that you will motivate someone else by what you are doing and how you are accomplishing it so they can do the same thing. The more you talk about your methods and process the more it re-enforces what you should be thinking about.

Mental weight loss has to be focused on daily, all day long and as often as possible. The more you are talking about the system and how you are losing weight the better and when you have others excited that helps you to drive even harder with your mental weight loss.

How incredible would that be for you? You start losing weight and in turn you help others to lose weight? You create a cycle that is not only healthy for you but, for others as well. What an incredible legacy to build that you will be able to help others with what I am helping you with.

There are so many people that are looking for leadership and help to get somewhere better. They are looking for shining examples that will guide them to greatness and by you helping them it will encourage you even more all the while losing weight and feeling great. Be proud of what you are going to accomplish and share it with the world. You could start a big movement with this and help so many people along the way.

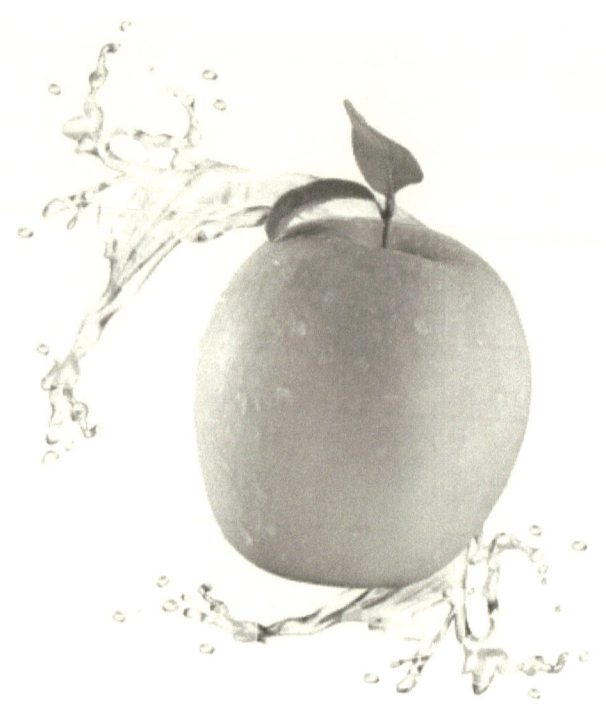

Chapter 4 – The Placebo Effect

You've got to say, I think that if I keep working at this ana want it badly enough I can have it. It's callea perseverance. ~ **Lee Iacocca**

Have you ever heard of someone taking sugar pills believing that they would do something for that person and because they buy into the idea that the pill they are taking will help them in some way? Don't you think that we all need what is called a placebo? Is it really hard to believe that we need to believe in things so we can focus our attention off of the problem at hand?

A placebo is a substance having no pharmacological effect but given merely to satisfy a patient who supposes it to be a medicine. Now how can this have an effect big enough and long enough for there to be a definition after it? Another words, how can someone imagine something like a sugar pill or another kind of placebo help them in some way? How is this possible?

By now I am sure you can figure out what my answer is to this equation and that is the mind determines everything for us either by choice or experience. If your mind believes something is real or has a purpose then that is what will go on.

Have you ever noticed that two people could get the same cancer, have the same amount of time to live and yet one will live and one will die? If I can get you to hear anything I want you to hear me scream this because your mind is powerful and you can and will determine how healthy or unhealthy you will be.

So the placebo effect as I call it works even when you know something is a placebo. After all, why not give yourself a placebo to focus on? Why not start to use food or movement or whatever you determine to become your placebo?

Let me explain a little bit further about my theory in the hopes that you may understand how you can be more effective in helping yourself lose the weight you desire. I used many placebos to lose weight including foods that were previously not thought to be healthy for me.

When you eat or drink food and you feel they are unhealthy for you even though you eat them anyways you are telling yourself to store fat and put on weight because you are determining that outcome. So why not determine that they have other effects like fat burning, energy increasing and happy mood creator? Seem stupid or not logical? Well why not when you are always stressing out over food and have nothing but negative outcomes.

I have used water as a placebo, vitamins, food, drink and natural remedies as my placebos and still do to this day. I use this stuff as a reminder of what I want and that is to be healthier and keep the weight off or lose some weight. I create my own placebos and so can you if you will open up and believe in them.

I have shown others how to do this and I have seen it work in their lives. So far it has worked every time but I am sure that someone will fail at it but I believe that will only be because they do not believe.

My entire program revolves around you opening up your mind and believing in many aspects of my mental training. The more you can access your brain power, the more you will gain as a person and as a healthy human being. Weight loss lies in your head.

The bottom line to the placebo effect is that you have to believe in what you are doing. Choose what you wish to as I did but it is important that you really believe in it. My wife still laughs at me but the difference is now she stops quickly and now laughs at herself as she eats her chocolate for a fat burning activity!

Mindset Training

Most of what I teach involves mindset training. I believe that solid change in your life comes from re-wiring your mind and because of that we need mindset training to establish a new mandate for your life. Mindset training forces you to learn new behaviors and thoughts based upon what you desire and need.

I believe that most people become unhappy in life because they fail to do one thing on a regular basis and that is mindset training. I believe that they become too busy to stop and refocus their mind and when it comes to weight loss or healthy living, I believe the problem becomes even bigger. I believe most people forget to properly focus the mind on what they eat, the weight they want to be at and how they feel inside.

What you focus on in your mind you will make happen so why not focus on the ideal weight you desire. This is the first place to start because you need to understand the goal that you want in order to properly focus on it. Let's take a look at how we can do some mindset training for weight loss.

All day long you think about all kinds of things and it is up to you as an individual to determine what you think about. There is really only one exception to what you think about; if you do not control your thoughts your mind will take over. In order to work on our mindset we need to focus in on every aspect of our body, weight, health, energy, mind, spirit and more. Let's take a look at your mindset on food and train your brains what you should be doing with it.

First off, if you eat like I did and eat eight to ten times a day you will not be so focused on being hungry all day. Tell your brain to communicate with your body that everything is okay and you will not be starving your body nor will you be over indulging three times a day either. You will feed your machine as often as it needs in small settings.

This already is a huge new mindset as you are probably currently telling your brain to communicate with your body that you are starving or stuffed and neither one is a great conversation. Your stomach is always in a state of expansion or contraction and often is in pain from too much food or too little food. You need to remove the pain and any extra conversations you are having about any of these meal times.

Your day should not be about food, food, food. Yes there are times when food is fun and something to look forward to but, if you are focusing on it mentally three or more times a day other than deciding what to eat then you need to cut it out now. The more you carry on about food internally, the more you are going to show externally (i.e. Weight gain) Relax, eat eight to ten times a day and learn to think about other more productive things.

Once we are past thinking about food all day, your mindset training on your ideal weight can take place. Let's say your ideal weight is one hundred thirty pounds and that is what you have decided to make happen. I want you to close your eyes, look down at the scale and see the numbers 130 on the read out. See nothing else on the scale in your mind.

Now keep visiting this in your mind everyday like a hundred times a day. See your weight on that scale. Look down at your body and imagine what one hundred and thirty pounds will look like on you and focus on that all day long. Mindset training will be this easy if you will practice it and believe it.

Next, your ideal healthy life is you moving as much as possible. You must see yourself moving in your mind. Focus on your body working at maximum performance while you are walking, running, chopping wood or whatever you decide to focus on. Does not really matter as long as it is a real activity you see yourself able to perform and you tie the experience to your body. Remember that the brain tells the body what to do even when you are sitting in a chair.

Mindset training in my weight loss program comes from working out our mind all day long. There are no breaks, there are no repetitions like in weight lifting and then take a break. There is no hour at the gym and then go home because we will have to work hard to get the results we desire with our mind. Yes it is very powerful but, we have to make up for the lack of physical work out we are not doing. I want to make it very clear to you that weight loss is never going to be easy. I do believe there is an easier way than what you have been probably doing if you are anything like me yet still it is never easy. What my system does for you is makes losing weight easier.

We all let things slip away from time to time and really life gives us what we focus on. The problem comes in when we focus on something new then we tend to let something else go but, your weight and your health is just not one of those things you cannot afford to let slip away. Everything we do in life that is good is tied to a healthy life style. Everything diminishes when we are lugging around extra weight, feeling tired and are breathing heavy and sweating.

Excessive weight deminsihes your capability in life such as having sex to enjoying family time, working on projects, work, and vacations and on and on. Go ahead and get mad I said that entire statement but, at the end of the day you know what I am saying is exactly true. If you are struggling with your family I bet health has something to do with it (enjoying them) If work is a big downer and you hate your job I bet weight and fatigue have something to do with it. We are all guilty of allowing ourselves to let our focus slip from our health but the point I am making is that we really cannot afford to let this happen.

The good thing is that we can get the focus back and we can repair the damage or harm from the weight gain. We can become again what we once were if we will focus our attention daily to our ideal weight and health situation. Trust me when I say that I was in a bad place and I knew it. I also knew I had to figure out something quick and I did. Where I finally become smart was that I did not go back out and run myself into the ground. I focused so intensely everyday just as I am still doing today.

Natural Supplements

This book and program is not about being foolish any more than it is about eating poorly and not feeding your body the nutrition that it wants. Your body craves goodness in many forms and I believe the reason we resist things so much is either we do not like the idea of certain things (like dieting or exercise) or we do not understand the importance of it (like supplements and vegetables) so we just push them away instead of accepting them and utilizing them.

The first half of my weight loss was exactly as I have laid it out to you. I did not diet and I did not exercise. I did change many things and I did add some things into my body and routine and supplements are one of them. In fact, both my wife and I had started on taking them even before my weight loss starting in 2002 when my wife was hospitalized for a bad case of Chron's Disease. I then started taking them again in 2007 when I was diagnosed with type II diabetes.

Then one day I decided that I wanted to lose 100 pounds and get healthier than I had been since college and maybe ever. In the previous two times I started with natural supplements and vitamins and homeopathy type remedies both my wife and I had huge success. Both of us no longer have symptoms of our previous diseases and we had really started to feel great. Now that I wanted to lose the weight and had plenty of years of research on supplements and other natural remedies I knew that I needed to kick it up to an even higher level.

I will not get into each and every kind of supplement I take but, I would encourage you to do your homework on them. There are two supplements I will talk about because I believe they were and are a powerful placebo and have been awesome for my body. The first is Aloe Vera Gel Caps. We get them from GNC (not a paid endorsement – just the best deal and quality I have found) and they come in a brown bottle. I am not officially endorsing them but what I will tell you about Aloe is that as a supplement it not only heals cuts and burns and scrapes on the outside but, in my opinion does an incredible job on the inside of the body as well.

We discovered Aloe back when my wife was sick and we both have taken it in small and large quantities. I won't give specific quantities because I do not want to be held responsible for your choices but, we made sure we knew what we were doing and so should you. We have also told so many others about this over the years and they have seen similar results as we have. Again make your own choices but, I believe this is one of my secret weapons in my weight loss, health recovery and youthfulness.

The other supplement I have been taking is called Graviola and I get it off Amazon for under $9.00 a bottle. This stuff is incredible as well and has all kinds of benefits to it. This supplement has benefits from mood enhancers to possible healing benefits and more. Do yourself a favor and start to learn about what supplements can do for you and your weight loss and health.

The Conversations I Have Internally

Have you ever taken the time and realized the conversations that you are having daily internally? You are having them even if you are not paying attention to them. The problem is that even though you may not consciously pay attention to them you are listening to them sub-consciously. This can be a huge problem if the conversations are not good or the right ones for you.

Much about this book and the program is about the internal conversations you should be having daily. It is about programming the right information in and then focusing on them. I will not tell you everything I talk to myself about for fear you may think I am off kilter or a little funny. I will tell you that I am talking to myself all day and night long and making sure that the conversation is being monitored.

As I have stated before the conversations start before my feet hit the ground. I love starting off my day being grateful first of all as well as picture having my crew go through startup mode for my machine. I love picturing what my day is going to be like and talking it out.

I jump in the shower and the conversations continue. The conversations usually also get tied to visions as well but, not always. When I make my first small meal of the day and taking my vitamins and supplements I have more conversations. I talk myself through my day, my weight focus, how I feel and how I want to feel. I know that I must focus on what I want or I will not get it so I go through my entire check list daily. Here is a sample list of my daily check list I go through and add to it as needed:

1. How do I feel?
2. What is stressing me out and how to fix it?
3. What am I grateful for?
4. Am I having troubles with my relationships and how can I make them better?
5. Is my machine fired up and running at full capacity?
6. Am I focusing on food too much?
7. What do I need to do to feel stronger?
8. How can I improve myself today?
9. Do I feel angry about anything?
10. Do I need to forgive anyone today?

There are more but, these are the important ones and when I ask these questions I focus on the answers and carry on the conversations that I need in order to get the answers to these questions.

You have been told all of your life that talking to yourself is weird or unhealthy and answering yourself is even worse but, I say they are all wrong. If you do not have these conversations and participate in them then you are not going to be able to do what you really want and that is to live healthy and lose weight. Talk away to yourself and discover what you can learn and become.

If I am not in a physical conversation I am in an internal conversation and in fact even as I write these words I am carrying on. Talk and listen and answer and let your mind know what you want, work through problems and stress and find a way to get to where you can burn pounds without resistance.

Creating Visions in My Mind

I get asked a lot by people about creating visions and goals in my mind and how I do this particular activity. It often gets asked of me how I see something that is not there physically. I understand how some people can struggle with creating visions yet on the other hand we have been doing this kind of thing our entire life and never think twice about it so it does baffle me a bit.

How many of us have ever seen the Easter bunny, Santa Clause, the Tooth Fairy or God physically in front of us but, we can all see visions of them in our mind. Some have been planted and others have been created but, either way we create visions in our mind and this is just one powerful example of how you can create powerful visions in your mind if you can just remember your past visions.

What about when you were a child and you wanted something really special? What did you do about it? You persisted and you dreamed about it and you created the vision in your mind of you playing with it, holding it or whatever it is you do with it you saw you performing it. So what has changed?

You may not know exactly what something looks like but, with a little research you can get yourself going. What is important is that you can see yourself that way in your mind. After all, the saying goes that seeing is believing, right? If you can see yourself a certain way then the image is powerful. How will you see yourself five inches smaller and with less belly fat if you do not create the vision? Right now your body may be telling an entirely different story and if that vision is not pleasant then you will not focus right.

For me when I create visions, the visions themselves are affirmations of what I want and the confidence that they will occur. You might ask if I am able to create every vision I have that comes up in my mind. No because priorities change but, the majority of my visions come to fruition because I believe in them.

I also like to create accurate visions in my mind because the more specific they are the better my outcome. If I want to wear a size thirty four pants then that is my vision. I do not just vision smaller pant size. I actually see the size 34 tag as I pull them out of my drawer and slip them on. You must be very specific.

Visions are a story teller or future teller for the mind. Again, you are creating visions already even without you paying attention to them. A lot of people create doom and gloom visions and because of that you are receiving doom and gloom in real life. Change your visions and you will change your world

Happy Activities Equals Happy Life

One of the reasons I wanted to lose weight and get healthy was because I was doing less and less fun activities. When you are three hundred and thirty six pounds it is not easy to go out and do much of anything let alone "fun activities."

What defines fun for most people? This is a great question and one that I realized changed for me from when I was skinnier to when I put on all of that weight to when I took it all off and kept it off. The reason is that weight gain or loss changes how you look at things. When I was in shape rock climbing, hiking, softball and other things seemed like a lot of fun! Then I put on weight and sitting around relaxing, playing Tiger Woods Golf on the PS3 sounded better and lots of yummy food. Then I took the weight off and fun changed again for me.

The meaning of fun changes as well because when I was heavy the fun was not that great and often had consequences with them. Weight loss fun has more meaning, freedom and my outlook is so much greater.

Would you agree that what makes life so exciting is the possibility of the fun and enjoyment that you can get from it? The more fun that you can accomplish in your life, the better your outlook is on life. I know that holds true for me and struggling to have fun is not the same as having plain old fashioned fun.

The reason I am pointing this out to you is because you need to have more fun in life. You need to be free from the unhappiness of weight gain and obesity. You need to feel alive again and not lethargic and this will happen as you begin to improve your weight, your attitude and your pants or dress size.

Happy activities equal a happy life and the sooner that you can get back to there, the sooner your life is going to feel more complete. Weight gain is not fun and carrying around extra weight is tiring and depressing and I want you to feel better because I know I do. I want to share with you what it feels like to remove the chains of obesity and go out into the world freely and enjoy it.

- **Thinking Thin Moment:** Here is what I would like you to do right now. I would like you to think about a time when your weight was ideal and right where you wanted it. You felt great and weight was not a focus. What did you do back then? What activities do you wish you could do this very moment? I want you to focus on that for several minutes and enjoy the experience.

Fat Burning Activities

I understand that most of us hate to exercise and that the very thought of exercising makes us cringe but, we truthfully still need to work on fat burning activities. The first fat burning activity we work on daily is having our mind communicate with our body that we are burning fat all day long.

This activity is equated with everything you do throughout your day. I say some funny stuff about Thinking Your Way to Thin but, I absolutely believe it all. I burn fat walking and I burn fat vacuuming. I burn fat taking out the garbage and I even burn fat drinking water. It is that simple for me. I visualize the water just flushing out the fat in my system. You must see this and believe it.

Everyone in my house knows I am serious about this stuff and at first they struggled to grab on to it but, after a while they all have understood it and now even use it. They talk about what they are doing to burn fat and what food they eat that burns fat. If we believe in this fat burning activity mindset then we can tell the brain to send the signal to our body to get burning the fat. Along with eating constantly and everything else in this book, you can begin to take back the controls to your body.

There is still the option of light to moderate exercise and sweating away the pounds as well. I do not recommend it though until you start to understand how your mind plays into losing weight and not until you start to lose the pounds. Exercise is not inevitable but, the benefits of movement are great. I tried not to have it in my mind for the first 30 pounds but everyone is different especially if you have been taught exercise is the only way to go to lose weight.

Hold off on exercising or gaining more movement until your mind matures into this How to Think Your Way to Thin Process because I do not want the typical frustrations to leak into your mind. Exercise is great for you in moderation and as long as you are enjoying it. I hated it at my heaviest so I avoided it at all cost.

I concentrate on fat burning movement. What is fat burning movement? Any kind of movement that I do that I deem to be fat burning activities. I also like energy movement. What is energy movement? I think you are starting to get the picture.

A Side Note

Take a look at your diet and do an inventory of fruits and vegetables. If these do not make up at least 30% of your diet you should try and add more of them into it. Lemon is great in water and on chicken. I learned to eat broccoli and fresh spinach even though I previously hated them.

Eat more carrots and onions and garlic are so good for your body. Your body craves nutrients and goodness and starving it of these essential foods is a huge mistake. There are also capsules that can help with this as well. Give it a try and see what it does for you and your body as you may be very surprised the improvement that comes from bumping up your fruits and veggies.

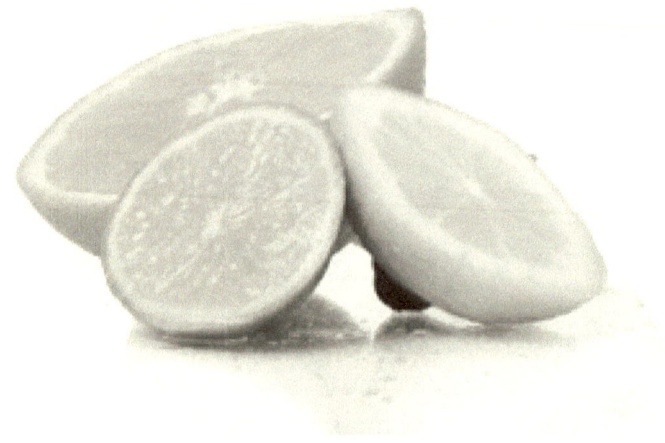

Chapter 5 – Thriving in Your New Body

The chains of habit are generally too small to be felt until they are too strong to be broken. ~ **Samuel Johnson**

Have you ever heard about the lottery winners who end up broke within a few years after winning the lottery? The reason that this situation occurs is simple really; bad with money before the lottery and you will probably be bad with money once you have it. The same holds true for losing weight as we have to get right before we get there or we will surely get ourselves into bankruptcy quick! Learn to be good with your weight now and not suffer later.

You have to become clear on how you are going to act as you make your way to your ideal weight and body size. This is important and I want you to take it serious right now. Remove old mindsets, feel great about your body, go out and have fun and love life to the fullest. I want you to focus on burning fat and repairing your body.

When you start to lose weight and I mean significant weight loss where you can see it in your face and your waist, celebrate and smile big. Share your success and let others know that you are a champion. Be energetic and let your new body thrive out in the open instead of hiding behind a baggy sweater or sweats. Go buy a few new clothes, pull out the old ones with dust on them that was once just an idea and dream.

It is also time to start having a casual attitude about things that once stressed you out. The new you is not hung up or obsessed with putting on weight or allowing others to stress you out. Be free I tell you and learn to let go.

You must change your behavior to lose weight. You must admit to your failures in order to correct them. You do not have to beat yourself up over them but, keep it real at all times.

As I began to lose noticeable weight I did something slightly wrong. I was almost in disbelief at one point. I admitted to what I was doing working but, kept moving on in my journey without acknowledgement. Ninety five pounds later I still was not totally clear what I had done. The pants sizes decreased and so did the shirts but, I really had no clue the amazing feat I was accomplishing.

You know what hit me the most about what I had accomplished? The pictures on the front of this book woke me up and I said, "WOW!" My family and I were looking through old pictures from 2006-2008 several months ago and we came across a folder that said Mom's Funeral. That in itself was hard to look at but, then we came across the picture with me holding her bible and I was blown away. I was huge in that picture but, more importantly I was now amazing as a few folders later on her computer was the other picture on the front of the book as well in the black shirt. Guess what? That picture is over 2 years old as well and I have lost more weight and am in even better shape than when it was taken.

I knew what I was doing was real and I knew I could succeed but, truthfully I had no idea how awesome the whole experience was until several months ago and that is why I wrote this book and created the program. What I had done was nothing short of amazing. Now I want you to feel what I did and experience what I have.

You will thrive in your new body if you are ready to prepare yourself ahead of time and start fresh. Give yourself the gift of life. Get ready for a new life and a new look. Chin up, mind strong and shoulders out.

Some have suggested that losing weight is simple; eat less and exercise more and no one needs guidance from some guy who wrote a book and program. Like somehow I am preying on vulnerable people but nothing could be further from the truth. First of all you are not prey or weak people. You are in need of guidance which brings me to my second point and that is like you I have tried and failed at losing weight. I discovered a formula that works and since I created it who better than to teach it to you. This is no different than a football coach teaching you his play book. This is not about me being right and you are wrong. Weight loss is not as simply stated by some who say eat less and exercise more because if it was that simple you would already be where you want to be right?

Losing weight is mostly mental and understanding how to properly set you up is essential to your success. My hopes is that this book sets you on the right course so that you can do exactly what I did.

What Do You Think About This Idea So Far?

By now the idea has to be winning you over or you will for sure going to struggle trying to succeed. I do not say this to put the wrong thoughts in your mind but, we are 98 plus pages in and if by now you are not grabbing on to this idea then you are going to have a tough time.

If you are struggling with this idea then ask yourself why you are struggling with it. Is it because it does not fit traditional methods? Are you struggling because you cannot see yourself like that thin body you used to be? Have you always been over weight your whole life? Wipe any worry out of your mind and start to look for reasons why all of this will work for you. Look for reasons why you like this idea and why it will work for you.

To achieve great success in anything you have to look for reasons why things will work. Looking for reasons why it will not work is mostly a waste of time because you will be right. Time better spent is on figuring out the reasons why it will work for you to accomplish the goal at hand.

This idea I have presented to you is very powerful and when it starts to work for you your mind will rapidly change. Towards the end of the book you will find the simple daily elements or the abc's of how to fully work this idea but, you need to understand this whole thought process first and foremost. The magic is in your mind and philosophies.

You might ask why smart people have not figured this out yet and why do I know it and next to no one else does? The truth is that some have started to figure it out especially in pieces. They have learned parts of it but, next to no one have put it all together as they should and as for the smart people, I bet they have it figured out yet they do not necessarily use it for weight loss.

I know the Special Forces have it figured out like the Marines. I have heard it called other names and applied in many situations but, for some odd reason when it comes to weight loss we do not believe it as much even though we have plenty of examples.

Let's not focus on why so few have discovered it and let's focus on the fact that you now have discovered it. You are going to start today to think your way to thin. You are going to use techniques that hardened Marines use.

What do you think so far? Do you believe that you can do this? Do you believe that you can use techniques with your mind that can help you to burn fat? Do you believe that you can speed up your metabolism mentally and naturally?

You see I believe that we have been searching for the fountain of youth for thousands of years and it has been here the entire time. Youthfulness lies in the mind first and the body is a natural after effect of your thoughts.

Have You Tried Growing a Garden?

One of the most gratifying activities I started doing a few years back was growing my own organic garden and not just because I was eating more vegetables and fruit but, because I was eating organic food that was healthier for me. I was also researching more about food and health and nutrition, was learning about safe ways to eliminate pests and bugs from my garden and because there is something really cool about growing things from a seed from your own hands.

Having my own garden every year is such a gratifying experience and every year I want to learn more and more all the while I am eating healthier and healthier. This activity lifts my spirits and pushes me to be more responsible for my health.

People tell me all the time how they wish they could grow a garden themselves but, they are too busy and have no time. What I suggest to you if this is your reply as well; when I have been working all day and I want a salad and I am out of tomatoes or onions or cucumbers I do not have to run to the store. I simply go out to my garden and I pick what I need. No trip to the store and I have no wasted time and my vegetables and fruit taste healthier and sweeter and chemical free.

Do not let the excuse that you have no time stop you from growing some or all of your fruits and vegetables and herbs. It really makes no sense. Also, every year we spend very little and eat so much goodness all the while saving a lot of money. Plus, very little goes to waste this way. When I shop at the store we are always throwing stuff out.

I love having more control over what I eat as there are so many bad things in our food these days especially processed foods and chemicals on our fruits and vegetables and herbs. Also when you run out you have to wait until you go to the store again for more but, not with your own garden. Go out and grab them when you need them. Freeze your own for the winter.

Overall, growing your garden is a great way to take charge of your health and it is a great way to contribute to your personal life. Even if you do not have much room you can still grow things like herbs or certain vegetables relatively easy. Pinterest is a great way to get ideas if you need some. All you have to do is just search gardening or vegetables etc. You will quickly see what I mean by all of the ideas and pictures that pop up.

Why Some People Live and Some People Die

Okay so the title is a bit startling but, I wanted to catch your attention. Growing up and my most of my life I thought that rich people had a better chance of pulling through disease or heart attacks or cancer because they had money. They could have surgeries, medicine or whatever they needed to pull through whatever they might be going through including prevention methods.

Today I believe something entirely different in the way of that idea and I do not want to get into this idea too deep because I believe it to be a whole book in itself but what I will cover is the aspect of money or no money and cure and prevention.

I believe many times that the reason some people die when they get sick is that they give up, give in or have a very negative outlook. I also believe that some just never truly fight and believe they are not going to pull through.

Do you think what I am saying is kind of wrong or harsh? There are so many examples of people who fight cancer and beat it and some who just fight harder and come out all clear. Then there are some who just lie down and die. Doesn't this sound familiar to you? Attitude determines everything maybe?

Almost 20 years before my Mother's death, she went to the doctors where the doctor told her to go home, lay down and she would probably live six months with the heart problems she had. She decided differently and made it almost twenty years. My Mother was a fighter and had determined she would not go out so easy. She would fight it, get into better shape, eat better and prove the doctor wrong and she definitely did just that.

The reason I bring this to light is because I want to drive home the point that there is a ton of power in your mind. What you think about will come about. You might say that people you know who died did not want to die and that might be true but, was death on their mind constantly at the end? I don't want to die is a much different thought than I want to live! Proper focus is so important.

Set your mind straight and you will see the results that you want. Over the years I have surely discovered how amazing the mind is. I have always received what I wanted one way or another. Whatever I have focused on I have received both good and bad. I wanted those things or I would have never focused on them.

Will you be the one who loses weight or who puts on weight? What will determine which one that you will do? Will you be the one who decides to stand up and believe it, declare it and live it?

Who Do You Want to Be?

When I looked down at my stomach one day way back I knew that I wanted to be something else other than what I had become and I believe early on I did one thing that was huge (no pun intended) that changed everything for me. I asked myself who I wanted to be. This is a question that is very thought provoking and can have a huge impact on you just like it did me.

When we stop asking high gain questions of ourselves, then we will stop the high achievement that we truly desire. I asked myself this question and then I went on a journey to discover the answer. As a person I knew who I was and was very confident in my nature yet I was struggling in my fat suit I had built for myself.

Something I should make clear to you is that even at three hundred and thirty six pounds I was still very active and was as strong as an ox yet that was no real consolation as I forgot who I wanted to be as a body. I just got up every day and had no real plan. Sure I exercised and tried to eat healthy but, no plan was in place. You must plan for a healthy and good body.

That is why this question that I posed was so important because it meant that I was ready to plan out who I wanted to be as a healthy body. I know had a chance to mold the body that I wanted and would no longer just get up every day without a plan and the end result is not only my body but, this book and course has been written.

Since asking that question just take a look at all that it has been accomplished. Because of that one question I have become healthy, lost one hundred and five pounds and I am now able to write this book to help thousands do the same.

That is how powerful questions can be especially with your weight loss.

- **Action Item*** I want you to spend several minutes alone in a quiet place and ask yourself who do you want to be? Create a vision in your mind that you would want to be. Create your own vision as everyone does not have to be a skinny model or a ripped body builder as this book is not about that idea. This book is about achieving the body you want to be healthy in. Create the vision, grab the vision and focus on the vision daily so that you will end up where you want to with your body and health.

How Should You Feel About Your Weight

My first piece of advice of how you should feel about your weight is to turn off the runway shows and tear up fitness and model type magazines (no offense to any of these outlets) because you do not need to look like any of these people. Skinny to you could be one hundred and forty pounds while it is ninety eight pounds to a fitness magazine.

If you want to be like those people in the magazines that is fine but, you will be creating some extra pressure on yourself. This pressure is fine as long as you can handle it and want it.

I use other people's visions all the time. If I want a certain style of house I go and look for one to create my vision so

109 | P a g e

another body you like is the same idea. I do not live in the mansion I want yet but, I still keep the vision alive in my mind as a focus marker.

Now to get back to the question at hand in the title of how you should feel about your weight, I will say that you should feel honest about what you want at all times. I always liked how I looked on one hand with the exception of how my clothes hung off of me but, I certainly did not like how heavy I had become. I liked my body except my stomach and chest. If you told me I was fat, heavy or obese I would have agreed with you.

Being overweight seems to be an emotional hot button for people. When people are overweight and you bring it up in any way they get upset, mad, and emotional as well as cry and even more. Why do you think this is the case? Do you believe that this emotional instability might be one of the very main reasons that weight loss is such an issue? If you can get so upset over words then maybe, just maybe the weight needs to go and you need to create your body type you have in your vision?

Emotions are a detrimental force that will work against your weight loss plans. If you cannot learn to control your emotions then how you feel about your weight is always going to be an issue and will more than likely control your outcomes. No matter where you are at right now you have to make peace with it because it is where you are at. If you think getting stressed and emotional about your weight is going to serve you then I would ask you how is being emotional working now and in your past.

I would imagine some of you are tearing up as you read this question and I do not ask it to get you crying but, I want to get you real with the issue. I see too many people that either cry and get emotional and upset (yes mostly you ladies) and others who get mad and defensive and irate (yes you guessed men, that is you) and it is like being frozen for them. They are too committed to the emotion and not the solution.

The fact is that you should not accept your weight gain and think it is okay or that you are beautiful the way you are but, you should also not feel embarrassed or ashamed either (I made this mistake). Be real with where you are and hold your head high. You are an awesome person and just because you have put weight on do not mean you are worth any less.

The beauty of being obese or over weight is that you can start over any time and get healthy. As long as you are alive you can reverse the effects of being overweight.

Play a Game and Have Fun

I knew that in order to lose one hundred plus pounds, I was going to have to work on not getting bored, frustrated and lose any motivation. After all, it had taken me a long time to put on the weight and taking it off was not going to be quick so I decided to make my mental weight loss into a game and have fun with it every day for having fun is life's ultimate prize here on earth.

Every step of the way you need to remember that attitude determines everything and because of that you need to make losing weight a fun game. You need to smile a lot, laugh, and enjoy the experience.

I remember that when I first started telling my family about my plans to lose weight and how I was going to do it they looked at me like I said I was going to fly to the moon. It made me laugh as I saw their reactions.

Then as time went by it became even funnier as they were in disbelief as to how I was losing the weight and yet all I was doing was mostly sitting behind my computer. The longer this went on the more challenged I was by how funny it was to me.

I went for months making all kinds of jokes and enjoying the experience with them as they were in disbelief over what I was accomplishing. This mental weight loss thing I was doing was great entertainment not only for me but, for my family as well.

I have learned that as a human being that if people are not having fun in life then they become a detriment to themselves. This occurs from small harms to large ones and everything in between. What that tells me is that if you do not have fun with losing weight then you will find a way to sabotage yourself. Do not let that happen.

Which brings me to another theory of mine and that is that average people often complain that other people sabotage them and hold them back and as much as I am sure there are bad people in this world, this is not really true. I believe that we often sabotage ourselves most of the time and right before the finish line.

You have nothing to lose by having fun except weight and the more fun that you have will help you to lose more weight. Go ahead and make it all a game while you lose the weight you desire and you will be smiling all the way to the mall for new clothes.

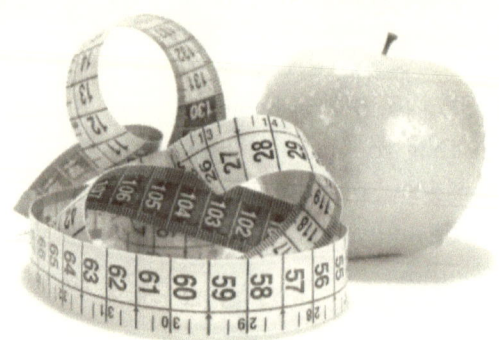

Chapter 6 – Daily Routine for Weight Loss

Take care of your body with steadfast fidelity. The soul must see through these eyes alone, and if they are dim, the whole world is clouded. **~Goethe**

Something I learned a long time ago as an athlete is that routine and repetition is the key to an elevated level in your success. You always hear the same thing from championship teams and that is

we practiced the basics over and over again until we could not get them wrong and then we perfected them. You losing weight are going to involve doing similar activities that will ensure your success. There is no need to look for big homeruns because all you really need is a bunch of base hits. People always think too big and complicated when it comes to weight loss.

Why is a routine so important with weight loss? The answer to this is that what you need to do is establish is a new discipline and new habits. Just because I am helping you to unlock mental weight loss does not mean you can work out when you feel like it! You have to establish a routine and make sure that you stick to it.

I have never done anything great in my life where I did not have to be in a solid routine to accomplish it. You need to be structured in order to change stubborn habits like over indulging with food, poor mindset, lack of motivation and other habits that you have been living long term.

Everything I have laid out in this book is one giant routine that you have to consciously decide to take on to become a new reality for you. If you read this book, jot down a few ideas and then try one of the ideas every once in a while then you will fail. I do not say that to be negative or wish ill will on you but, to make the point that success is going to come from discipline and an established routine.

Meditation and Yoga and Stretching

There is nothing that I have suggested that has not proven to work and as we march our way through this book that you will decide to fully engage in every one of these elements or ideas and use them to create a routine and new life style.

It is extremely important to have a peaceful time that allows you to work on your mind and body. I am not a yoga expert on any level but, I understand it enough to know that it is a very good tool for your health.

As far as stretching goes I believe that it is essential to living long and feeling good. All three of these activities really should involve stretching. I believe this is a secret to a long and fulfilling life which is combing stretch with a form of meditation.

As you get older, your body gets tighter and tighter. The tighter the body gets the harder it gets to move around and to feel great. Your body cannot operate as freely because of this situation going on. You hate to exercise or do not prefer to partake in it then I urge you at minimum to take on stretching daily (if not several times a day).

Next, as we get older I believe that our mind gets tight as well or closed off. Meditation will free your mind and help you to open up the possibilities in life and this can happen in a relaxed and peaceful state. Since both of these are very important to your health why not combine them into one activity?

Mental weight loss is about taking time for you and working on yourself. I am a personal growth and development guy and I learned the value of doing these types of activities many years ago and now that I have discovered how valuable it is in weight loss I study it even more intensely than ever.

Our life experiences are made up every second and every minute we are awake regardless if we can walk or not, if we get out of bed or not or if we act on our goals and dreams or not. If we are willing to subject ourselves to new ideas and give it everything we have then we can create the life experiences that we really want.

Give one or all of these a shot. They really are all related but do have their own disciplines and I urge you not to turn away from them. Do you need them? No, you could skip them but, they are not hard on your body and the value of them is tremendous. Give yourself a gift as you think your way to thin.

Removing Toxins from Your Body

Have you ever owned a fish tank before? If you have and you were good at taking care of it then you learned about something very valuable in doing so. What you learned is that you need to have the water as neutral as possible in order for the tank environment to be good or you will lose lots of fish. The reason I am giving you this example is that your body is a lot like that fish tank because balance is really important.

The body over time can become very acidic and also full of bad toxins. The first place I suggest that you start is flushing out the body with plenty of hydration. Water is your friend especially if you can get filtered and alkaline water.

If you have been on antibiotics in the past and especially for any period of time or multiple times, I suggest (in my opinion) that you flush your body of these because they tend to make you toxic and cause more harm than good.

I try as much as possible to use natural, homeopathic type solutions as much as possible. I am not advocating not doing as your doctor says unless you feel it is best for you and of your own opinion. What I do say is that adding anything into your system that is not natural and foreign is never a great idea. Doctors tend to suggest prescriptions to maintain an illness and not a cure.

I suggest that you spend time studying natural ways to cure disease and ailments and find supplements that will work with your body naturally. Find ways to flush the body of toxin and acidity.

Over the last fifteen years my wife and I have found many ways to cleanse the body and remove prescriptions drugs and other medicines and have freed ourselves of diseases that require lifelong medicines and debilitating side effects. There are no guarantees in life but all study shows that a cleansed body is a healthy body.

There are also a ton of natural fruits and vegetables, herbs and other naturally grown plants that will help you with cleansing the body and bring you back to neutral.

Stay Away From Stressful People

Nothing will make you want to run to comfort foods or a glass of wine quicker than stressful people in your life. I cannot point out enough that you need to take inventory right here, right now and start to remove stressful people from your life like a spring cleaning of the millennium. Fill up a big cardboard box, write free on the outside of it and put it out to the curb with all of those people who bring stress and drama to your life.

Never make excuses for where you are at or what you have done. Let's face the facts that besides ourselves nothing else can get us doing harmful things to ourselves like the people in our life. We trust them enough to be close to us and then we lower our guard. Ultimately it is up to you to allow whatever may go on but, they can bring you stress quickly which will bring you a thicker midsection out of nowhere.

Why is this even possible? Simple; we do not pay enough attention to what stressful people do in our lives and we often make excuses for how they act. They are around us and in our lives and we get fed by then every day. At first you pick up on it here and there but, after a while you just over look it until you explode one day from all of the tension.

This is not a people bashing section but, instead is a protect your weight loss section because if you do not watch who you spend time with you will surely pay the price.

Stress can crush you quick and ruin all of your hard work. When you have stressful people in your life, they usually are focusing on themselves and are oblivious to what they are doing to you. They live this way regardless if you are in their life or not and I am not saying you need to remove them immediately but, if they will not cooperate then you very well may have to remove them all together.

If I believe that I have a potentially good relationship with someone toxic with side effects I will have a talk with them and try and get them to knock off what they are doing. If after several attempts they persist on what they are doing then I remove them from my life one way or another. I cannot afford to take the chance with my health with someone who is selfish.

People who bring stress to your life often do not guard their mouth either and can be detrimental to your mental weight loss. Ultimately you are going to have to toughen up and not let anything side track your success but, up front I urge you to keep away these people in your life even if you just go on a vacation from them for a while. I guarantee you will find hitting your goals so much easier.

When I was at my heaviest of three hundred and thirty six pounds I was surrounded by people who stressed me out. I never really showed it too much on the outside but, on the inside I was beside myself and frustrated by their actions and full of stressful pressure. I understand first-hand about what these types of people can do for your health. I know doctors love to tell you to reduce your stress but they never give you any clue how to do it. That is why I am giving you this huge secret on how to reduce stress. Remove stressful people and you are more than half-way home.

Mental Weight Loss Partner Training

When I decided to lose weight mentally I had no one to help me with what I was doing after all I was inventing my own system. What I would suggest doing once you have a plan in place is to recruit someone to help you with your goals by recruiting a mental weight loss partner for training.

Accountability is paramount to any goal or dream that you have and you want to ensure that you accomplish it. I would caution you though to find someone who will elevate you, match up to where you want to go and will never give in to tough times and fold on you.

You can find someone who wants to work this process with you or they can be your mental weight loss coach. No matter what you decide to do be cautious of your choice. The obvious is that this weight loss system is all mental and you do not want the wrong person working with you. They need to encourage you and remind you and most of all keep you accountable to the goal.

If you find someone you want to partner with get them a copy of this book right away so they can read it and get on the same page as you. Ask some interview questions and make sure that your choice is solid upfront so that you do not pay for it on the backend.

Your mental weight loss partner should be that one person who can help you get back up if you fall down and understands how to properly motivate you.

There are Over 50 Names for Sugar

As far as I know there are over 50 names for sugar and who knows there may be even more. I think if we are going to set ourselves up for success with our weight loss then we should get a grip on our sugar intake and learn a little something about what has happened to our food.

Do not panic as I have not changed my position on losing weight but, I have never hesitated to eliminate things that make it tougher for me to accomplish my goals and sugar is defiantly an enemy of great weight loss.

So I told you what happened to me in February of 2007 when I was told I had type II diabetes. First I was depressed and even a bit scared when I was diagnosed; after all I had just lost my mother a few months before due to complications from the disease.

Next, I was angry about my new position and all that I was saddled with having to do to take care of this unwanted disease. I was on medicines that made me dizzy and sick and schedules to keep etcetera.

Then I decided I was not going to settle for this sentence that was placed on me. I did what I do best and that is I started to research for a solution. It was slow at first but, here is where a huge moment made so much clear for me and it has never left me since. I learned that sugar had over 50 names for it. For example here are a few of them so you will understand how crazy this is. Sugar, brown sugar, barley malt, caramel, corn syrup, fructose, glucose, fruit juice concentrate, dextrose and dextran to name a few. This is very deceiving and if you are trying to lose weight then you need to cut out some or all of these. This was the first thing that really shocked me and taught me something very valuable.

The next thing that I learned was that often times (more times than not) when food says non-fat it usually means they have substituted the fat for sugar. Does this even make sense other than to confuse you into buying their fat-free food that will become fat from all of the sugar?

If I had learned nothing else then this would have been enough for me. These two things are a sure sign that we are being over loaded with sugar and it is a major epidemic. The food items that include sugar are through the roof and most people do not even have a clue about it. Check out what I am saying and see if you can find any of the sugar names in the back of the book is in any of your food especially food that you thought had no sugar like milk for instance.

The last thing I will bring up here is processed food and that is full of preservatives like salt and yes there is even sugar in a lot of it. Check your labels and cut out even 35% of your sugar intake and watch what happens to your waistline.

I knew early on that what I had learned was going to be very powerful and not because I was going to have to cut out some sugar so I could lose weight but because it opened my eyes and focus on things that are working against me. I did not know better before but, since learning this I had a responsibility now.

The Power of Prayer

I do not know what your spiritual preference is but, mine is God and being a Christian and I believe heavily in the power of prayer. Prayer time is not only essential to my faith but, is also a great time to reflect on my life and ask God to help me be better in my life.

I believe that prayer is a time to be calm, at peace and focus on my relationship with God and because of that I give it a lot of respect like turning off my phone, focusing on my time with God and listening. When I was my heaviest I thought I was near death and it drove me closer to God and my faith. I believe God was trying to wake me up to what I needed to do about my weight.

I have faith in prayers and I believe it saved me from a catastrophic ending. I thank God that clarity came to me in my time with him in prayer as I struggled at the beginning.

What set me free one day and helped me to relax was my faith. My faith in God taught me to have faith in my mental weight loss. I must believe even when there is no physical presence involved.

The power of prayer is very powerful for many reasons and I hope that no matter what you believe in that you can appreciate the analogy or the understanding that I learned from my time in prayer.

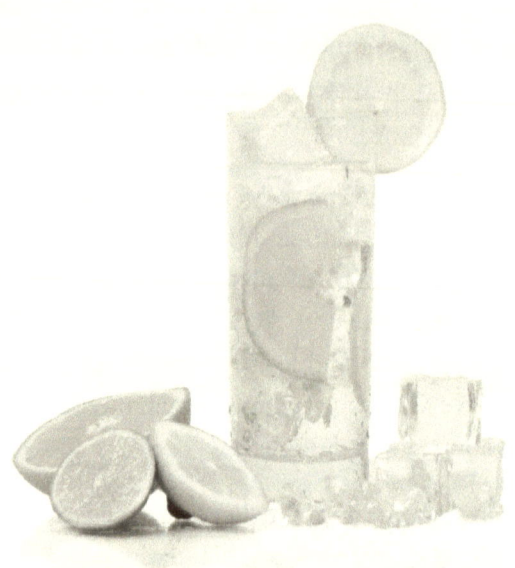

Chapter 7 – My Thinking My way to Thin Step by Step Process

The good Lord gave you a body that can stand most anything. It's your mind you have to convince. ~ **Vincent Lombardi**

Step 1: Before you get out of bed every day do a few very powerful things; be thankful for the greatness in your life and focus on getting your body moving, working efficient and burning fat before you let your feet hit the floor.

Step 2: First thing in the morning drink a cup of lemon water even before you brush your teeth. Toothpaste has sugar in it and so does mouth wash and doing this first will trigger fat storing. Instead burn fat, prepare your body and kidneys and drink water throughout the day. Get into the shower and use the time of getting ready for your day as a time to reflect on what you want with your weight loss.

Remove any doubts, negative thoughts sand see the inner workings of your body as a well-oiled machine.

Step 3: Before you put any food in your mouth always make sure that you are focusing on telling your brain that what you are eating is fuel for your body and that it is to burn fat. Scream inside of you that fat burning will commence immediately.

Step 4: Visualize mentally all day long your new body, the mental exercise you are doing just as if you were doing it physically (i.e. Visualize that you are doing pushups, crunches, and running activities). Focus on the ideal weight that you see on your mental scale.

Step 5: Take your vitamins and natural supplements and tell your body that these are essential to your weight loss and helping your machine hit peak performance.

Step 6: Maintenance your mind every hour on the hour and remove limiting beliefs, negative thoughts and increase your new mentality with positive affirmation.

Step 7: Check in with your accountability partner, write in your journal or spend time in prayer. Do all of these often enough that you feel like you are not alone in this journey and that you can work out your thoughts.

Step 8: Eat every couple of hours so that your body is constantly being fed fuel and energy. Remove feeling bloated or weighed down and get rid of feeling hungry. The more you feed your body the more you will speed up your body. I am not talking about increasing the amount of food but, take the same amount of food and break it down into more small meals.

Step 9: Find little ways to get movement, stretching, Yoga or meditation or even a walk to the end of your driveway. These are low exertion activities with high impact on your mind and body.

Step 10: Remove stressful people from your life, enjoy the good relationships that you have, laugh, have fun and do not stress or obsess on things.

Step 11: Learn about food, nutrition and supplements. Grow a garden if you can and eat organic. Remove small things from your diet that you know for a fact is terrible for you. Make them gross in your mind and remove all temptations.

Step 12: Eliminate 50 names of sugar from your diet and try and remove as much processed foods as possible.

Step 13: Eat the food that you want and have no guilt. You must change the way you see food. If you need comfort pick up a book, go for a walk, watch a movie or anything else that does not relate to food.

Step 14: Create a routine and stick to it. Make sure that you have reminders everywhere of what you are trying to accomplish. When you feel stuck, remember that this is only a feeling and it is temporary. Your routine and discipline will carry you through as long as you commit to them.

Step 15: Pray often and seek God's strength as well as his vision of you. Use this time to be at peace and one with God.

Step 16: Mindset determines everything and because of that you must focus every minute of every hour and never let up. Take your mindset and elevate it to an outrageous level. When your mind is optimal the body will follow. It has no choice because the mind is in charge of the body.

Step 17: Be thankful for the body that is already yours before you go to bed. Live a life of gratitude each and every day and never worry about what you have already done. Only focus on what you can do because you have been given the opportunity to start fresh and determine your own future.

Simple Daily Plan

If you think about it clearly planning your day is extremely important to weight loss and healthy living. Depending on what you do for a living you may need to plan for proper meals, drinks and more.

When I was my heaviest I was always out and about on sales calls and did not plan very well for my nutrition. I ate out a lot at restaurants, fast food, convenience stores and more when I was hungry or thirsty. I felt like it was a privilege since I was working so hard and long hours. The privilege should have been that I took the time to better care for myself and eat better.

Planning gives you the ability to guide elements in your life to come out the way that you want. Without planning you end up with whatever happens. Things may come out good for you and then again they may come out horrible. Planning is the great equalizer

I suggest planning out a few weeks at a time at minimum. The more detailed your plan the better off you will be. Plan ahead for travel, long meetings or work days and time you will spend alone with your thoughts.

Simple daily planning could be a very powerful piece you have been missing in your life when it comes to weight loss. Most people fail to plan and when it comes to eating. If you are eating because you are starved and desperate you are making a huge mistake for two big reasons; your mind knows you are doing wrong and your body can feel it because the food is usually not healthy.

When Will You Know It Is Working?

When will you know if it is working for you? In the beginning you will have to have faith and just know it is working but, you should start seeing results immediately in the way you feel mentally and then within 30-90 days depending on your situation you should start to see physical results as well. There is no magic to exactly when it will happen yet it will happen.

Like everything in this book, I suggest that you do not focus on the results of weight loss upfront or really ever. I understand how you may feel and you want to look and feel better now and because of this I will assure you that if you will stay with this focus long term you will see the results.

There is no weirdness in this process except the fact that I have lost over a hundred pounds in a way that is different to everyone out there who tells you how to lose weight. Everything else has been perfectly designed for you to do what you need to do to lose weight.

What I suggest is that you believe in it right from the beginning and that you believe in it working from the get go. Faith plays a huge part in my weight loss plan. Do not give in to temporary feelings or emotions. You are going to feel great and soon you will look great as well.

It took me over a year to lose my weight and I never let down. I could have lost the weight faster but, I was not interested in straight weight loss. I was interested in life style change that would serve me a life time and you should be too.

You are almost to the end of this book and the time is nearing where you will have everything that you need to get yourself mentally fit for weight loss. Where you need to go from here is to a new life. You must take what you have learned and push on and make sure that you never let down.

It is time that you believe in yourself and get started down the road to your ideal body weight. Change your mind around these new ideas and learn to relax and enjoy life more. I know anyone can do this program and I have sure seen the results from it over and over again with myself and others who I have taught.

Maybe you should go window shopping and start to dream about the new clothes you will soon be able to wear. Maybe think about a great vacation that you want to go on once you are healthier and lighter.

I want to thank you for reading this book and I pray you will put it to use. I want you to succeed and I want you to be happier and more fulfilled in your life. I want you to feel incredibly healthy and get those pounds to melt away without disrupting your entire life.

For me I am off to work on sculpting my body a bit now that I am able to again. I lost a whole person with my mental weight loss and unfortunately I lost some muscle too so I am focusing on that and my total gym workouts. I am also focusing on working with my wife and clients on How to Think Their Way to Thin which has turned out to be a very pleasant surprise.

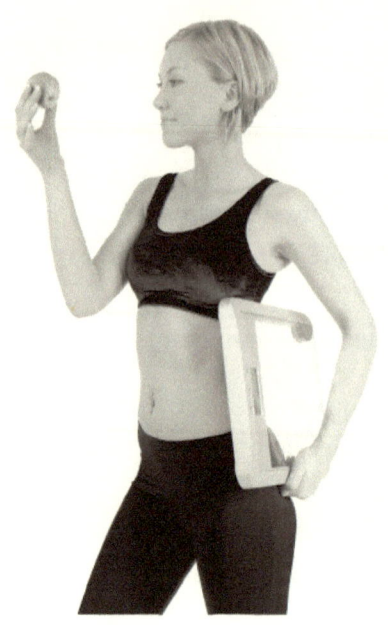

Chapter 8 -Summary and To Your Greatest Success

You have now arrived at the end of the book and it is now time to take the journey to your healthiest live ever. I wanted to just give a brief summary on where you started, what you learned and what you will do now that you have read this book.

Before starting this book your weight has been an issue and you have been feeling frustrated and worrisome about the idea of losing weight. Food is an issue for you and you stress out way too much about everything you put in your mouth. You seek out comfort in food and comatose yourself at times to escape.

You learned habits growing up from your family in regards to eating habits and because of that you have been living unhealthy. You have too many stressful people in your life and stressful situations.

What you learned is that you must be thankful every day and have gratitude for your life. Your body is no longer a body but a well-oiled machine that requires start up daily, maintenance and routine and is the best focus for you daily.

A machine is tough, strong and powerful and can get the job done.

Eating is for fat burning, power and nutrition and not to over indulge with. You are focused and vision what the food is doing for your body all day long. Be strong, be fit and be wise on your journey.

You have learned to eat several meals throughout the day because three meals a day is too much for your body to process and keeps you hungry in between. This idea involves more work on the front but, far less on the back end for you and your body. Feeling bloated is horrible and you will not do this to yourself any more.

You have discovered that you have to keep yourself mentally fresh and fit as the key to weight loss lies in your mind. You will work out mentally and visualize your ideal weight, clothes and how you feel.

The best thing I can tell you is that attitude is everything so make sure you pick a good one to use. Weight loss secrets are all about you and your attitude towards food, life and mental health. Do not pay attention to the critics because they will steal your happiness away. You get to be what you see in your mind so make sure no one else paints that picture for you.

Best wishes to you and I am hopeful that you will take this encouragement from me and drive yourself to the top. Lose the weight you desire, get healthier, feel better and enjoy your life.

About The Author

"A strong positive attitude will create more miracles than any wonder drug." ~ *Patricia Neal*

This book encapsulates everything that the author stands for in life. Robert Kintigh believes in the ordinary person doing extraordinary things harnessing the brain power and heart inside of them. Robert believes in second chances and the comeback story in life. Robert believes that the mind is a powerful tool and that harnessing every single electrode and thought is extremely important to obtaining the success you desire.

For over 23 years Robert Kintigh has been an entrepreneur in a variety of industries where he has made a name for himself with mindset training, leadership, sales training, employee behavior modification and personal growth and development to name a few.

His writing skills set him on a journey of helping individuals and companies with important aspects to growth and development. His passion for writing makes for dramatic ideas presented in unique settings and genres.

Robert has been married for 20 years to his wife Sallie and has three children. Robert is building a legacy for his family through his writing in the hopes one day they will provide a window inside his soul for his family to learn from.

Professionally Robert hopes to help people to remove the limiting beliefs they have placed on themselves and show them that the power they seek to accomplish anything is already inside there with them. Mental focus is powerful and amazing.

Robert wrote this book after struggling to lose weight for over three years and discovered that the way everyone else talks about weight loss did not make a lot of sense to him. As usual he was willing to sacrifice himself to put to the test if this method was viable. After three years of testing and implementing he decided the time had come to launch it to the world.

Robert's first book called The Lies We Tell Ourselves was launched a year ago and since then he has written several other books that have been on the best sellers list on Amazon. His first book was a personal growth and development book, as well as a success manual for those of you who want to understand the secrets to success. In his first book Robert provided real life examples and situations in order for his readers to learn from as he did not want to have to sacrifice others for them to learn from.

In this book How to Think Your Way to Thin Robert has designed a weight loss program to go with the book as well as other products to support his writing. You can go to www.truthmastery.com and check out what Truth Mastery has to offer and click on the link in the navigation to How to Think your Way to Thin.

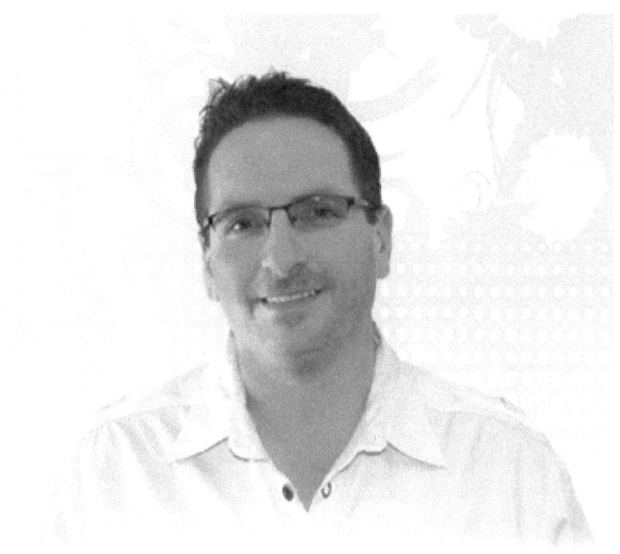

50 Names for Sugar Glossary

1. Barley malt

2. Beet sugar

3. Brown sugar

4. Buttered syrup

5. Cane juice crystals

6. Cane sugar

7. Caramel

8. Corn syrup

9. Corn syrup solids

10. Confectioner's sugar

11. Carob syrup

12. Castor sugar

13. Date sugar

14. Demerara sugar

15. Dextran

16. Dextrose

17. Diastatic malt

18. Diatase

19. Ethyl maltol

20. Fructose

21. Fruit juice

22. Fruit juice concentrate

23. Galactose

24. Glucose

25. Glucose solids

26. Golden sugar

27. Golden syrup

28. Grape sugar

29. **High-fructose corn syrup**

30. Honey

31. Icing sugar

32. Invert sugar

33. Lactose

34. Maltodextrin

35. Maltose

36. Malt syrup

37. Maple syrup

38. Molasses

39. Muscovado sugar

40. Panocha

41. Raw sugar

42. Refiner's syrup

43. Rice syrup

44. Sorbitol

45. Sorghum syrup

46. Sucrose

47. Sugar

48. Treacle

49. Turbinado sugar

50. Yellow sugar